GROW TALLER AFTER PUBERTY
EXERCISE ROUTINE HAND BOOK

STEPS TO TAKE TO GROW TALLER AFTER PUBERTY AND COMMON MISTAKES TO AVOID

DENNIS RANEY

ISBN - 9798665944319
Growtallerwithshinlengthening.com
First Printing 2014
Disclaimer and Terms of Use: Although every precaution has been taken in the preparation of this digital book, the publisher assumes no responsibility for errors or omissions. Nor is any liability assumed for damages resulting from the use of the information contained.
Your reliance upon information and content obtained by you at or through this publication is solely at your own risk. The author assumes no liability or responsibility for damage or injury to you, other persons, or property arising from any use of any product, information, idea, or instruction contained in the content or services provided to you through this book. Reliance upon information contained in this material is solely at the reader's own risk.

CONTENTS

PROLOGUE

When faced with the challenge of being short in stature, you may try everything to add an inch or two to your height. Some go as far as risking their lives with surgery.

Those who can't risk surgery either try natural methods or give up altogether.

At some point in time, I belonged to the bracket of those who tried natural methods, failed at a point, persisted, and I was fortunate. The secret to this success is investing time, being consistent and persistent. If you have limited time, then your chances of success are limited.

Bear in mind that your final height is determined by both natural and environmental factors and the two, work hand in hand. Natural Factors include genes and illnesses. You may have the genes, but with poor nutrition or diseases, you may fall short of your maximum genetically predetermined height.

On the other hand, much as you manipulate the environmental factors like nutrition and exercises; you may not grow more than 3 inches taller than your genetically predetermined height unless you opt for surgery. So, your genes contribute a lot to your final height. To understand your maximum height potential, look at all your close relatives.

For instance, you may have short parents with taller grandparents or aunts, uncles and cousins. In which case, your chances of being tall are higher. Manipulating the environmental factors may give you a chance of being taller. My parents are 5'4" and 5'7" yet my uncle and cousins on father's side stand between 5'11" and 6'2".

This may have contributed to my success with using this particular exercise routine. So, if you're looking to creating yourself a grow taller exercise routine, this guide may be of great help. Based on more than four years of try and error, I share with you the steps you need to take to be successful and the many mistakes I realized which you should avoid. As you'll see, it's an easy to follow yet efficient exercise guide and if you're still in puberty, you will find tips for maximizing your growth potential

CHAPTER 1

HORMONES THAT INFLUENCE BODY GROWTH

Growth reflects a complex interplay of hormones, environmental influences, and genetic factors. The pulsatility of growth hormone *(G.H)* secretion under physiological conditions is controlled by a complex regulatory system primarily exerted by their hypothalamic neuroendocrine hormones that is; Growth Hormone Releasing hormone *(G.HRH)*, somatostatin (G.HIH) and Ghrelin.

G.H.R.H, is the principal stimulator of G.H synthesis and secretion while somatostatin is a potent noncompetitive inhibitor of the release of G.H and modulates the pituitary G.H response to G.HRH.

Human Growth Hormone (H.G.H)

A lot will be said about human growth hormones so what exactly is H.G.H?

Human growth hormone is produced by the pituitary gland located deep inside the brain just behind the eyes, and it stimulates the growth of muscle, cartilage, and bone.

It's made throughout a person's life time but is more plentiful during youth.

H.G.H instigates growth in children and plays an essential role in adult metabolism.

Scientists first isolated H.G.H in 1956. Three years later, N.H.S (National Health Service) doctors began to use it in the treatment of children suffering from stunted growth to help them grow.

Most G.H is secreted during the first 2 hours of sleep and after exercise. Under normal conditions, more G.H is produced at night than during the day.

In people of all ages, G.H boosts protein production, promotes the utilization of fat, and interferes with the action of insulin, to raise the blood sugar levels. G.H also increases levels of insulin-like growth factor-1 (IGF-1).

Therapeutic use

G.H is available as a prescription drug that is administered by injection. G.H is prescribed for children with G.H deficiency and others with very short stature and used to reverse muscle wasting in AIDS patients.

It's also approved to treat adult G.H deficiency — an uncommon condition that almost always develops in conjunction with significant problems afflicting the hypothalamus, pituitary gland, or both.

The diagnosis of adult G.H deficiency depends on individual tests that stimulate G.H production. Simple blood tests are useless at best, misleading at worst.

H.G.H has also been promoted as an anti-aging treatment Because of the importance of the H.G.H to the body's biochemistry.

Adults with bonafide G.H deficiencies benefit from G.H injections. They enjoy protection from fractures, increased muscle mass, improved exercise capacity, and are at a reduced risk of future heart disease.

Potential side-effects

Despite its broad range of therapeutic application, there is a price to pay.

Up to 30% of patients experience side effects that include fluid retention, joint and muscle pain, carpal tunnel syndrome *(pressure on the nerve in the wrist causing hand pain and numbness)*, and high blood sugar levels.

Excess H.G.H in the body can cause acromegaly.

acromegaly is a disease where the hands become spade-like in appearance as they get bigger and facial bones grow causing the face to change shape too.

The jaw becomes larger with spaces appearing between the teeth because of this, and the eyebrows become more prominent.

The tongue enlarges and the skin becomes coarse and oily. Organs of the heart, liver, and kidneys will also undergo excessive growth, leading to potentially life-threatening problems - like cardiomyopathy, a disease of the heart muscle where the heart loses its ability to pump blood and, in some instances, the heart rhythm is disturbed leading to irregular heartbeats.

There's also an increased risk of cancers due to the abnormal growth of cells.

Growth Hormone Releasing Hormone (G.H.R.H) also known as Growth Hormone Releasing Factor (G.H.R.F) or somatocrinin.

Growth hormone-releasing hormone is a hormone produced in the hypothalamus and cleaved (split) to generate the prime factor known as somatoliberin, which acts to stimulate G.H release from the pituitary gland.

In addition to its effect on growth hormone secretion, G.H.R.H also affects sleep, food intake and memory.

Insulin-like growth factor 1 *(IGF-1)*

Is a hormone produced in the liver and other organs in response to growth hormone and can be retarded by under nutrition.

IGF-1 is produced throughout life. The highest rates of IGF-1 occur during the pubertal growth spurt and the lowest during old age.

IGF-1 is the primary mediator of the effects of growth hormone.

Once growth hormone is released into the bloodstream, it stimulates the liver to produce IGF-1.

IGF-1 then stimulates systemic body growth and has growth-promoting effects on almost every cell in the body, especially skeletal muscle, cartilage, bone, liver, kidney, nerves, skin, and lungs.

In addition to the insulin-like effects, IGF-1 can also regulate cell growth and development, especially in nerve cells, as well as cellular DNA synthesis.

Protein intake increases IGF-1 levels in humans, irrespective of the total calorie consumption.

A synthetic analog of IGF-*1 (mecasermin)* is used for the treatment of growth failure.

Somatostatin *(also known as Growth Hormone Inhibiting Hormone).*

Somatostatin is a hormone produced principally in the nervous and digestive systems. The primary function of somatostatin is to prevent the production of other hormones and also stop the unnatural rapid reproduction of cells — such as those that may occur in tumors.

It regulates a wide variety of physiological functions. The hypothalamus is a region of the brain that regulates secretion of hormones from the pituitary gland which is located just below it.

Somatostatin from the hypothalamus inhibits the secretion of G.H by the pituitary gland. It's also produced in the pancreas and inhibits the flow of other pancreatic hormones such as insulin and glucagon. The pancreas also secretes it in response to many factors related to food intakes, such as high blood levels of glucose and amino acids.

Finally, it acts locally in the gastrointestinal tract to reduce gastric secretion of gastrointestinal hormones, including gastrin and secretin.

Chemically altered equivalents of G.H.I.H are used as a medical therapy to control too much hormone secretion in acromegaly patients and other endocrine conditions, as well as treating some gastrointestinal diseases and a variety of tumors. Because it's an inhibitor, somatostatin is essential

to balance hormone levels in the body and stop the effects of overproduction of certain hormones. G.H inclusive.

Thus, somatostatin levels that are too low can cause the problems associated with high levels of other hormones.

Growth hormone, in particular, can be problematic. However, this is a rarely reported condition.Excessive somatostatin levels may be secreted as a result of an endocrine tumor known as somatostatinoma. This tumor produces the hormone independently. The result is extreme suppression of the hormones inhibited by somatostatin.

An example of this is the suppression of insulin secretion from the pancreas leading to raised blood glucose levels *(diabetes)*.

Ghrelin

Derived from *"Ghre"* which means grow and *"relin"* which means release, ghrelin was first isolated from the rat stomach in 1999 by Kojima and colleagues.

It' s a gastric peptide that increases appetite, glucose oxidation, lipogenesis ***(the metabolic formation of fat)*** and instigates the release of G.H.

Ghrelin is produced and released mainly by the stomach with small amounts released by other organs like the heart, lungs, lymphatic tissue, kidney, adrenal glands, thyroid gland, pancreas, gonads, and the brain.

Ghrelin is suppressed by intake of nutrients thus it's normally secreted when the stomach is empty, and its secretion ceases when the stomach is full.

It acts on hypothalamic brain cells both to increase hunger, increase gastric acid secretion and gastro intestinal motility to prepare the body for food intake.

Ghrelin acts by targeting the arcuate nucleus ***(A collection of neurons in the hypothalamus of the brain)***, from where growth hormone releasing hormone neurons provoke G.H secretion.

How Age Plays A Role in Growth Hormones Release by The Brain

Spontaneous growth hormone secretion rates and secretory patterns were studied in a group of normal pre-pubertal children, adolescents, young adults and older adults by determining the concentration of growth hormone in plasma samples obtained at 20-minute intervals over a 24-hour period.

Pre-pubertal children secreted growth hormone only during sleep and not while awake and had a mean secretion rate of 91 µg/24 hours. *(µg denotes micrograms.)*

Adolescents secreted growth hormones both during awake and sleep periods and had a mean secretion rate of 690μg/24 hours.

Secretion rates in young adults *(21 to 41 years)* averaged 385 μg/24 hours.

Growth hormone was secreted during both awake and asleep periods but the number of secretory episodes was less than in adolescents.

In older adults *(42 to 62 years), the* total 24-hour secretion of G.H decreased and approached zero in three out of five studies.

These data clearly demonstrate an age-related change in the spontaneous secretory rate and secretory pattern of growth hormone.

WAYS TO MAXIMISE GROWTH HORMONE RELEASE

1. Weight lifting

Researchers divided women into two groups; one group did upper body training and the other a total body strength-training workout.

Some of the participants used lighter weights and high reps *(up to 12 reps before failure)* while the other used heavy weights *(up to 8 reps before collapse).*

The researchers measured the growth hormone levels of the participants before and after.

The women had more growth hormone in their blood after the workouts and levels were higher after using heavier weights.

In another study, researchers from Japan documented a transient rise in growth hormone in 16 participants after a high-intensity interval training session.

The participants pedaled an exercise bike at 85% of their V02 max *(maximal oxygen consumption)* for one minute with 30 seconds of rest between each set.

They completed 10 sets total. So, strength training, using heavy weights, and high-intensity exercise seem to boost growth hormone short term.

2. Get quality sleep for 7- 9 hours on a daily basis

The most considerable secretion of Human Growth Hormone occurs at night during the first two hours from the onset of sleep when you attain deep sleep also known as Slow-wave sleep though lower peak secretions continue throughout the night during sleep.

When Y. Takahashi and Daughday *(Washington University School of Medicine)* set out to monitor growth hormone secretion patterns during sleep at night, subjects included 8 young adults *(4 men and 4 women)* and the following was observed;

a. There was a significant rise in G.H concentration in the blood within 90 minutes after the onset of sleep.

b. The rise in G.H secretion was gradual, the initial rise detected 20 minutes to 40 minutes from initiation of sleep.

c. Some individuals attained peak G.H secretion by 40 minutes sooner than expected while others took much longer to attain peak G.H secretion.

d. It took between 39 to 165 minutes to attain peak G.H secretion though the average time was 70 minutes.

e. G.H concentration levels were high for 1.5 to 3.5 hours before slowly returning to baseline level.

f. G.H secretion patterns were reproducible throughout the night with sharp rises and falls though the initial peak secretion was the highest.

g. Those who had interrupted sleep or who were awaken for 5- 26 minutes, 2.5 to 3 hours from initiation of sleep and after attaining the first peak secretion never attained another peak secretion when they returned to sleep while those who had interrupted sleep for as long as 2-3 hours attained another peak G.H secretion when they returned to sleep.

h. When the onset of sleep was delayed, peak G.H secretion also delayed.

3. Consider Intermittent Fasting

Intermittent Fasting is restricting your food or calorie intake for a specific period during a given day usually 16 to 24 hours but can be extended if you wish.

You may take water or sugar and calorie-free beverage during this time.

As discussed earlier, ghrelin is a hormone released whenever food is anticipated and it is partly the reason why we feel hungry.

In other words, it's likely a conditioned response that prepares the metabolism for an influx of calories.

It's not necessarily the case that whenever the stomach is empty, ghrelin is released rather, it's released because food is anticipated which partly explains why first thing in the morning, we feel less hungry yet we've just gone 7 – 10 hours without eating anything.

Therefore, if you have fixed meal times, ghrelin secretion will peak at specific times when food is anticipated during intermittent fasting and declines after ingesting nutrients.

However, taking water does not affect ghrelin levels in any way and ghrelin levels don't remain elevated even when you don't eat.

They gradually return to basal levels after about 2 hours.

A study that was published in the European Journal of Endocrinology *(2002)* aimed to investigate how fasting results to elevated levels of G.H secretion among humans.

10 healthy men aged between 20 to 28 years fasted from day 1 at 12:00 hours until the end of the study, on day 4 at 20:00 hours.

Fasting rapidly induced a diurnal ghrelin and GH rhythm that was not seen in the fed state.

The changes in ghrelin concentration levels in blood during fasting were followed by similar changes in serum GH concentrations, indicating that ghrelin is the driving force of increased GH secretion during fasting.

4. Oral Ingestion of Amino Acids / Proteins.

Amino acids are the building blocks of protein. Akram *retal,* classifies them as follows;

Essential	Non-essential	Special
Lysine	Cysteine	GABA
Methionine	Tyrosine	DOPA
Valine	Serine	Citrulline
Tryptophan	Alanine	Ornithine
Isoleucine	Asparagines	Taurine
Histidine	Aspartic acid	
Phenylalanine	Glutamic acid	
Threonine	Glycine	
Leucine	Hydroxylysine	
Arginine	Proline	

GH secretion can be promoted by oral administration of various amino acids including arginine, methionine, phenylalanine, lysine, and histidine.

Leucine and valine seem less potent, whereas isoleucine does not seem to affect plasma GH concentrations.

In one study, 13 healthy male adults *(aged 18–40 years)* ingested a mixture of essential amino acids together with 200 ml water within 1minute after fasting for 10 to 12 hours.

After oral ingestion of 5 - 9g glutamine or arginine, plasma GH concentrations increased 2- to 4.5-fold higher in comparison with time controls.

Meanwhile, a combination of ARG and LYS increased plasma GH concentration 3 to 8-fold.

The rise in GH concentration started approximately 30 minutes after ingestion and peaked approximately 60 minutes post ingestion.

In contrast, oral ingestion of aspartic acid or cysteine did not affect GH concentrations.

5.High intensity interval training/ Exercising (chaos training).

High intensity interval training/ exercising *(H.I.I.T/E)* implies alternates between intense bursts of activity and fixed periods of less-intense activity or even complete rest.

For example; sprinting as fast as you can for one minute and then relaxing for two minutes.

Other examples of H.I.I.E include stair climbing or walking up hill.

A study from the *Dept. of Physical Education, Loughborough University, UK: 2002* aimed to compare 30 second all-out sprints to 6 second all-out sprints.

The participants did just one set of this all out-sprint and then H.G.H levels were monitored closely for 4 hours after the single sprint. *Here are some highlights…*

- Metabolic responses were greater after the 30 s sprint than after the 6 s sprint.

- The highest measured mean serum H.G.H concentrations after the 30 s sprint were more than 450% greater than after the 6 s sprint.

- Serum H.G.H also remained elevated for 90-120 min after the 30 s sprint compared with approximately 60 min after the 6 s sprint.

In a pilot study that aimed to test the hypothesis that high-intensity interval exercise significantly increases growth hormone, 5 young physically inactive women aged 21 – 25 years sprinted vigorously for 30 seconds without a break, before resting 4.5 minutes to recover.

The rate at which G.H was secreted within 12.5 hours was much greater and a single bout of this kind of H.I.I.E was enough to trigger the G.H secretory response.

How Chaos training Triggers G.H Release

For G.H secretion to be triggered with chaos training, you have to work out the muscles hard and fast enough to the point when muscle movement is almost impossible which is known as the lactate threshold.

It's the point when the muscles are too exhausted.

When muscle tissue contract intensely for a long period, the blood circulation system starts to lose ground in circulation of fresh air *(necessary for energy release)*.

In these circumstances the breakdown of sugar is changed to lactic acid.

As the lactate is created in the muscle tissue, it oozes out into the blood stream and is distributed around our bodies.

If this situation continues, our body performance reduces and the muscle tissue wears out very quickly.

This point is often calculated as the lactate limit.

The point when muscle is fatigued to the point of almost failing to move voluntarily.

The lactic acid is not responsible for the burn in the muscles as you intensely work out, but the hydrogen ions released as the lactic acid leaks out.

It's the high concentration of lactic acid in the blood that triggers G.H secretion.

CHAPTER 2

FOODS TO EAT TO MAXIMIZE BODY GROWTH POTENTIAL

Puberty occurs earlier among individuals who are well nourished throughout childhood and for those who have not experienced significant illnesses.

You need to consume a healthy diet with plenty of fruits and vegetables, and rich in nutrients like protein, zinc, calcium, and iron.

Cow Milk

Drinking cow milk during childhood is strongly linked to a child's growth and development.

However, non-cow milk like soy and almond milk is sometimes preferred by some parents because of its potential health benefits but such milk contains less protein and calcium compared to cow milk.

Thus, non-cow milk may not have the same impact on a child's growth like cow milk.

In a 2017 study published in the *American Journal of Clinical Nutrition* that aimed to establish whether there's a link between non-cow milk consumption and lower height in childhood, 5034 healthy Canadian children participated in the study.

There was a dose-dependent association between higher non-cow milk consumption and lower height.

For each daily cup of non-cow milk consumed, children were 0.4 cm shorter.

And 3-year-old children who consumed three 250ml cups of cow milk everyday were 1.5 cm taller than their non-cow milk drinking counterparts.

Another study on American children found that adult height was positively associated with milk consumption at ages 5-12 years and 13-17 years.

Milk contains calories, protein, and calcium, among other nutrients, and bioactive components such as insulin-like growth factor-1 *(IGF-1),* all of which may facilitate bone growth.

Some people question whether your body can digest IGF-1 through the intestinal tract.

However, animal data suggests that IGF-1 is indeed absorbed through the intestines and is biologically active.

IGF-1 is a hormone that promotes cell division and growth. However, its levels decline with age.

While IGF-1 is necessary for growth in children and teens, it may not be good to have higher levels as you age.

Clinical data indicates that in adults, more elevated IGF-1 levels are linked to an increased risk for cancer.

According to the Physician's Committee Responsible for Medicine, taking milk with lower IGF-1 will be less risky.

Either get milk from farmers that do not treat their cows with rBG.H *(Recombinant bovine growth hormone)* or Check the product for a label that says "rBG.H free" or "rBST free." RBG.H is a synthetic hormone commonly injected into cows in the commercial dairy industry to increase milk production.

RBG.H has sparked controversy and questions regarding the safety of drinking milk from cows treated with this hormone.

Cows treated with this hormone tend to contain higher levels of IGF1. Foods labeled certified organic are always rBG.H-free.

Other animal protein foods

The quality of protein is a function of the availability of amino acids it supplies.

Some protein sources such as animal products contain all of the essential amino acids.

Meat, poultry, fish, eggs, and dairy are all considered complete proteins.

If you consume two to three servings of these foods a day, you will meet your daily protein needs.

According to *Donald K. Layman* of The American Journal of Clinical nutrition, various protein

sources may exhibit different effects on bone metabolism.

Some, but not all, studies have found that animal meat *(including poultry and fish)* as a protein source is associated with higher serum levels of IGF-1, which is in turn associated with increased bone mineralization and fewer fractures.

However, potential health concerns do exist from a diet of protein consumed primarily from animal sources due to high intakes of saturated fats and cholesterol.

With a proper combination of sources, vegetable proteins may provide similar benefits as protein from animal sources.

If you're vegetarian or if you do not want to eat animal meats, soy and Quinoa a plant-based seed that is often called a grain are also complete proteins and a healthy option.

Besides quinoa and soy, proteins from plant-based foods are typically considered incomplete proteins because they only contain some of the essential amino acids.

Beans and legumes, nuts and seeds, grains, vegetables, and fruits are all incomplete proteins.

Combining two incomplete protein food choices in order to get all of the essential amino acids may help.

For instance, brown rice and beans will make a complete protein meal.

You may consider fruits like; Avocados, Guavas, Blackberries, Bananas, Jackfruit, Apricots, and Kumquats.

And vegetables like; Sprouted Beans including soy, Peas & Lentils, Lima Beans, green peas, Cooked Succotash, Kale, Broccoli, white cooked mushrooms, quinoa and Cauliflower.

Whey

Whey is the transparent liquid part of milk that remains after milk coagulates.

whey proteins are separated and purified from this liquid using various techniques to produce whey.

proteins in form of powder, concentrate or isolate which are popularly consumed by athletes.

Whey is a complete protein and all of the constituents of whey protein provide high levels of the essential and branched chain amino acids.

A 3-year clinical study of 342 healthy men and women 65 years of age and older also found that those who consumed the most protein and were supplemented with calcium experienced the most significant improvement in bone mass density, and most of the protein consumed was animal protein.

Low protein intake impairs both the production and action of IGF-1 *(Insulin-like growth factor-1)*.

IGF-1 is an essential factor for longitudinal bone growth, as it stimulates proliferation and differentiation of chondrocytes in the epiphyseal plate, and it's also essential for bone formation.

It can be considered as a key factor in the adjustments of calcium-phosphate metabolism required for healthy skeletal development and bone mineralization during growth.

Vitamins Necessary for Body Growth

Vitamin A

Vitamin A is essential when it comes to bone formation. Vitamin A is necessary for proper growth and development of our bodies.

It directly aids in growth by improving cell division and differentiation of many different types of cells.

According to the National Institute of Arthritis, musculoskeletal and skin diseases vindicate that vitamin A is essential in regulating the processes that keep our bones growing healthy.

Sources;

Vitamin A is found in most animal livers, fish like salmon and tuna, hard boiled eggs, and vegetables like carrots, kale, and cooked sweet potatoes.

Fruits rich in vitamin A include mangoes, passion fruits, cantaloupe, guavas, papaya, and watermelon

Vitamin D

Vitamin D is essential for the absorption and use of calcium and phosphorus by the body. It's necessary for the formation and health of bones, teeth, and cartilage.

Peak bone mass is usually achieved by 30 years. Therefore, physical activity and obtaining the recommended doses of calcium and vitamin D in adolescence and young adulthood will ensure peak bone mass.

Sources;

There are two forms of vitamin D; - D2 is found in some foods and D3 is produced within the body when the skin is exposed to sunlight.

10 to 15 minutes of sunshine, three times a week is enough to build the body's requirement of vitamin D.

Dietary vitamin D2 is found naturally in egg yolk, tinned fish, cod and halibut liver oils.

Vitamin D is also added to some foods. In the UK, margarine has to be fortified with vitamin D by law. In the United States, milk is fortified with vitamin D.

Vitamin K

This is an essential component in the body's normal blood-clotting process and plays an indispensable role in maintaining bone health.

Most vitamin K is produced by micro-organisms in the intestine and is stored in the liver.

Minerals that facilitate growth

Calcium

Calcium is essential when it comes to bone architecture and is required for deposition of bone mineral throughout life.

99% of the calcium in the body is stored in bones and teeth.

Sources

Dairy products, such as milk, cheese, and yogurt. Green leafy vegetables – such as broccoli, cabbage and okra. Soya beans, and sardines when eaten with bones.

Zinc

Zinc is a micro-mineral needed in the diet on a daily basis, but only in minimal amounts *(50 milligrams or less).*

When the effect of zinc supplementation on growth velocity was assessed, it was established that zinc supplementation increases growth velocity over a 12-month period.

Zinc plays a role when it comes to hormonal mediation by participating in;

a) Growth hormone synthesis and secretion.

b) The action of Growth Hormone in the liver.

c) Somatomedin-C production (Somatomedin C is another name for insulin-like growth factor 1 - IGF-1).

d) somatomedin-C activation in bone cartilage.

In addition to these multiple functions, zinc also interacts with other hormones somehow related to bone growth such as testosterone, thyroid hormones, and insulin.

sources

pumpkin seeds, beef, chicken, Cashews.

Fruits like; Apricots, Peaches, and Avocados.

Vegetables include; spinach, Palm Hearts, lemon Grass, cabbage, green Peas and mushro

CHAPTER 3

EFFECTIVE EXERCISES FOR BODY GROWTH AFTER PUBERTY

1. INCREASING HEIGHT IN THE TORSO.

There're three main ways to increase height in the torso.

A. Stretching exercises

B. Abdominal exercises

C. Thickening the spinal disc.

A. STRETCHING EXERCISES.

Stretching the torso can contribute to your upper body height in a number of ways.

First of all, back movement generally promotes the delivery of nutrients to spine, keeping the discs, muscles, ligaments, and joints healthier.

Thus, although speculative, it's possible that the various positions held by the spine during the stretching sessions retard disc degeneration by increasing the ability of nutrients to diffuse into the disc there by increasing the spine length.

Secondly, the stretching and positioning of the spine that occur during yoga exercises is believed to decrease the gradual disc degeneration that occurs with age.

It is also suggested that the constant tension and compression of the disc during stretching exercises stimulates the synthesis of growth factors by the fibrocytes and chondrocytes residing in the disc and prevents their degeneration.

Finally, in a study to investigate the impact of distraction, *(a type of mobility technique that we can incorporate into our stretching routines in order to create more 'space' inside the joint complex)* on spinal disc regeneration, the following was established;

i. 28 days of compression in rabbit disc caused degeneration via MRI study.

ii. 28 days of distraction/stretching regenerated the disc.

iii. Distraction/ stretching results in disc rehydration, stimulates extracellular matrix gene expression, and increases numbers of cells.

iv. Disc distraction/ stretching enhances hydration in the degenerated disc and may also improve disc nutrition via the endplates.

B. INCREASING SPINAL DISC THICKNESS.

The vertebral column or spine usually consists of 24 articulating vertebrae separated by Inter vertebral discs *(or inter vertebral fibro cartilage)* which lay between adjacent vertebrae in the spine, and 9 fused vertebrae in the sacrum and the coccyx.

Inter vertebral discs or spinal discs are the spongy material that lie between adjacent vertebrae in the vertebral column allowing the nerves to run between each bone segment and they are cartilaginous in nature.

Just like other cartilages, the intervertebral discs have no blood supply.

The required nutrients are seeped through from circulating blood by a process called osmosis and diffusion from the bone marrow across the cartilaginous endplate.

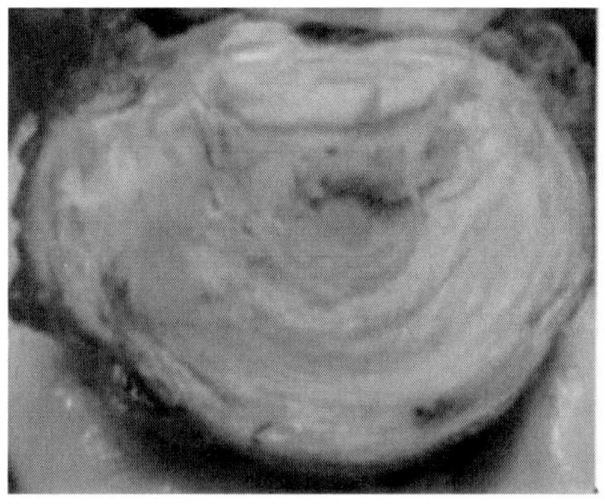

Collectively, the discs account for approximately between one third and one quarter of the total spinal column length interjecting the back bones from the top to the sacrum.

There are approximately 23 discs in the spine; 6 in cervical, 12 in thoracic, and 5 in the lumbar region.

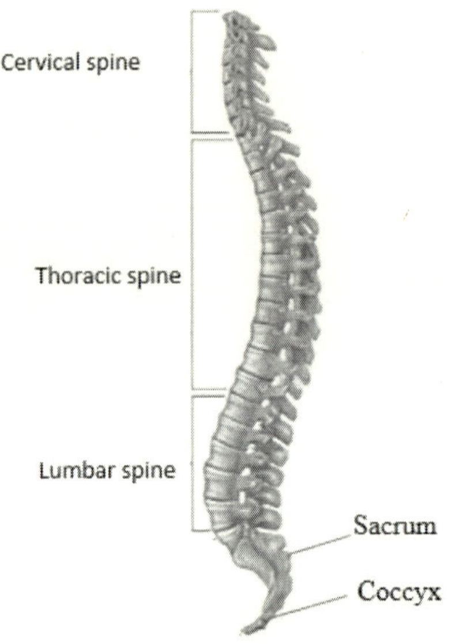

The discs in the lumbar region of the spine are approximately 7-10 mm thick. Inside the outer fibrous ring of the disc, is gel-like center, *(nucleus pulposus)*.

Disc degeneration is partly a result of the nucleus pulposus dehydrating thus limiting the ability of the disc to absorb shock.

This general shrinking of disc size is in part the reason why humans become slightly shorter as they age.

By age 40, approximately 25% of people show evidence of disc degeneration at one or more levels and signs of disc degeneration are apparent on scanned images in over 60% of the population after 40 years.

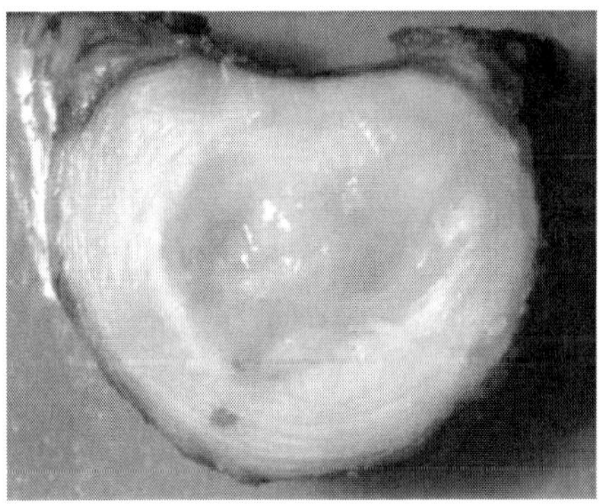

A disc made from cartilage has a typical thickness, of around 9 millimeters *(depending on which section of the back).*

There are 22 notable discs in the back of reasonable thickness.

Adding just a few millimeters of thickness to each disc will add typically around 3 - 5 inches of aggregate height.

Ways to increase spinal disc thickness

1. Sitting in backward slouched position

(propped slouched sitting)

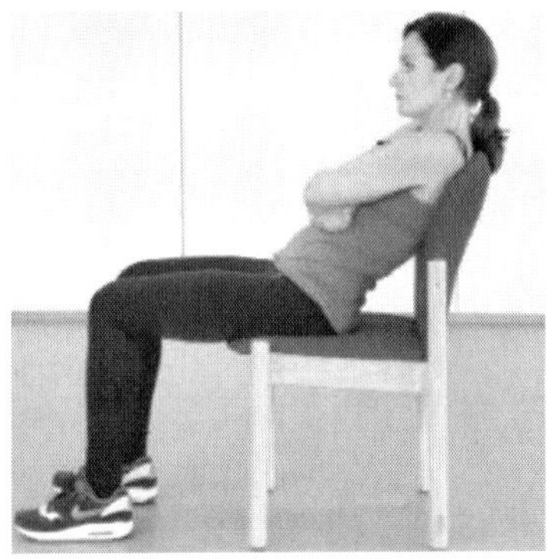

Sitting upright or in a forward slouched position is generally associated with increased pressure on spinal discs thus a reduction in spinal height.

Adams and W. Hutton *(1983)* suggested that fluid is squeezed out of the intervertebral discs much faster when one assumes a bent position.

When you sit with the back extended, it has the opposite impact and thus, it increases spinal height.

The reduction in inter vertebral disc pressure is attributed to the transfer of the load to the back rest.

In a study that aimed to investigate the impact of propped slouched sitting on spinal height after a period of trunk or torso loading, 40 subjects aged between 18 and 35 years both men and women participated.

Initially, the subjects sat upright on the chair edge, then slouched backwards and accepted support from the backrest against the mid/upper thoracic region as illustrated in the above image.

The subject's hands rested on a pillow placed on his/her thighs and variation of head position was minimized.

The subject then underwent loaded upright sitting with a 4.5 kg bag secured on each shoulder for 5 minutes.

The subject underwent a further 5 minutes of upright sitting without load to further reduce spinal height.

A digital stadiometer with the subject in the seated position was used to measure the entire spinal height.

The subject then underwent intervention propped slouched sitting for 10 minutes before taking measurements for the entire spinal height again.

There was a significant difference in spinal height before Propped Slouched Sitting and post propped slouched sitting *(from 883.61 mm to 885.56mm)* after just 10 minutes.

The increased spinal height with intervention propped slouched sitting posture suggested that after a period of trunk loading, such posture leads to rehydration of the lumbar intervertebral discs

2. Keeping the body hydrated

The spinal disc consists of two parts: The outer cluster of rings made of collagen called annulus fibrosus.

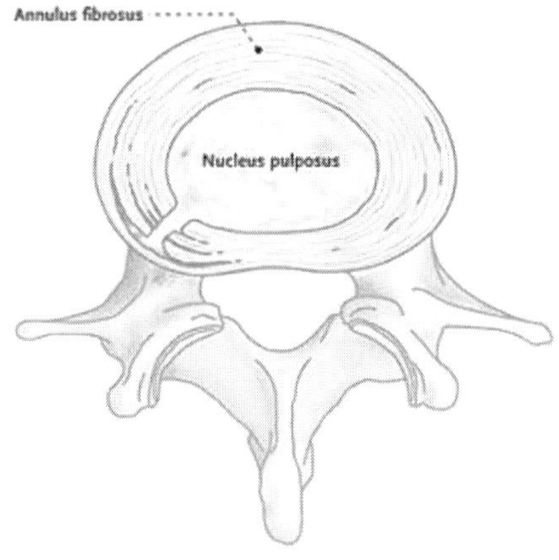

And inside the ring, is a gel- like substance called the nucleus pulposus which consists of 80 – 85% water.

Day to day activities like walking, sitting and lifting heavy loads like back packs significantly seep the water from the disc so, the disc keeps rehydrating as long as there's enough water in the body.

However, if the body is dehydrated, the disc will generally begin to shrink.

Besides reducing your disc thickness and overall torso height, this will adversely affect the spine health.

Once the gel- like substance *(nucleus pulposus)* which acts as the shock absorber shrinks, the entire load will be directly applied on the outer ring sometimes leading to chronic back pain.

So, most health experts recommend taking at least 1 to 2 liters of water every day. Not at once but throughout the day.

3. Supplementing with glucosamine sulfate and chondroitin sulfate.

Glucosamine and chondroitin sulfate are commonly used as food supplements to treat osteoarthritis *(A condition where the protective cartilage that cushions the ends of your bones wears down over time).*

To test the potential of the supplements to rebuild degenerated spinal discs which are also cartilaginous, in 1999 a 56-year-old man who complained of chronic low-back pain which existed for more than 15 years, volunteered to be moderately physically active by playing tennis during his free time.

On top of such moderate physical activity, he took capsules every day for the first 9 *months (two in the morning, one in the evening).*

Then 2 capsules *(in the morning)* for the remainder of the two – year period.

Each capsule contained 500 mg of glucosamine and 400 mg of 95% low molecular weight sodium chondroitin sulfate.

The patient felt a gradual improvement of the range of motion and functioning of his back, with less pain starting about 6 months from the date of his first supplement intake.

At the end of the 2 years period, his back felt stronger and more flexible and was capable of withstanding heavier workloads without pain.

Apart from this improvement, the overall physical condition of the patient remained unchanged during this period.

And most importantly, the patient experienced no adverse effects of these supplements.

A magnetic resonance imaging was performed at the onset of the pain and after one and two years of supplementing.

After oral intake of glucosamine and chondroitin Sulphate for two years, an increased water retention *(and less bulging/protrusion)* in the partially degenerated discs was observed.

4. Lying on an inflatable cushion or spine arcing device

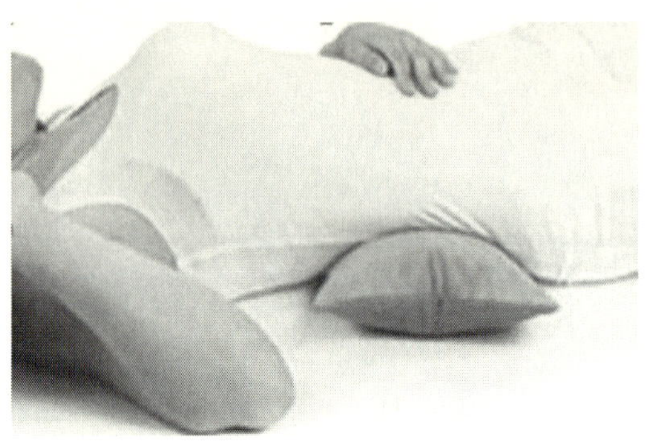

In an experiment that aimed to assess the impact of supine hyperextended posture on disc rehydration, 10 subjects aged 23 – 30 years lay in a supine position then an inflatable lumbar support/ cushion was positioned under the lumbar spine *(right under the peak of the spine curve)* for10 minutes to hyper extend the spine.

Measurements were taken before and after.

The average amount of height gain after 10 minutes in the supine hyperextended posture ranged from 2.766 mm to 7.66mm.

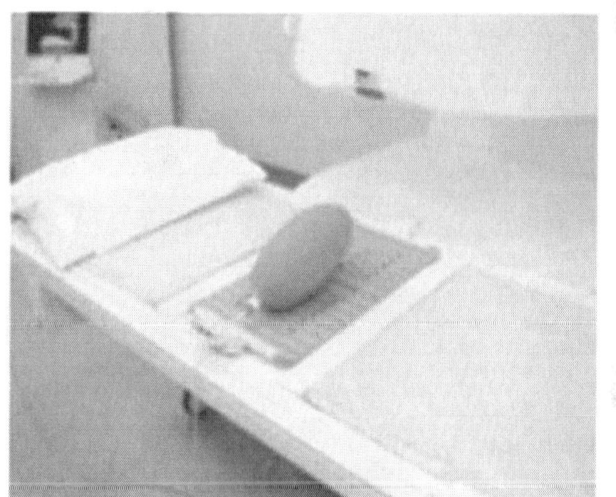

Inflatable cushion used in the experiment

C. ABDOMINAL WORKOUTS.

Abdominal workouts will stabilize or increase your torso height in three ways;

1. When the abdominal muscles are weak, the spine is not properly supported which leads to changes in body alignment or slouching.

This is because it's the back muscles especially those that run from the lower back to thoracic region *(The erector spinae and multifidus muscles)* that play the vital role of keeping the spine in position and with stand any forces that may lead to spinal disc compression like gravity thus keeping the spine in an erect position.

Slouching will definitely make you appear a couple of inches shorter.

2. Weaknesses in abdominal muscles may also result in compression of joints around the lumbar spine or the bottom portion of the spinal column which affects your spinal disc height and overall height.

3. Finally, Strong abdominal muscles will effectively carry the weight of your body and bones-thus taking some of the unnecessary pressure off your spine.

2. INCREASING HEIGHT IN THE LEGS

Increasing height in legs is quite tricky especially if you've passed the puberty stage but it's not impossible because I managed to do it, there are individuals who did it as you will read later and you too can do it if you're steadfast.

There are three ways you can successfully increase your leg length.

A. Cycling with a raised seat

B. Using ankle weights

C. Doing plenty of jumps every day.

A. CYCLING WITH RAISED SEAT

This is one method I endorse simply because I successfully used this method to grow my shinbones by approximately 2.5 inches over a period of 3 years.

Some fail with this technique but to increase your chances of success, first you need to do whatever it takes to increase G.H in the body and enough has already been discussed about how to achieve this.

That's one crucial factor many either disregard, don't know or miss out.

Others use protein powders as you will read under success stories but I never used supplements, so I have no comment.

If you always mind what you eat and focus on only what's essential for body growth, there will be no need for supplements save for the nutrients that are poorly absorbed by the body.

How to use cycling with raised seat

If you are starting out, raise the seat by quarter an inch then when you achieve the quarter gain in height, you may take it to half an inch.

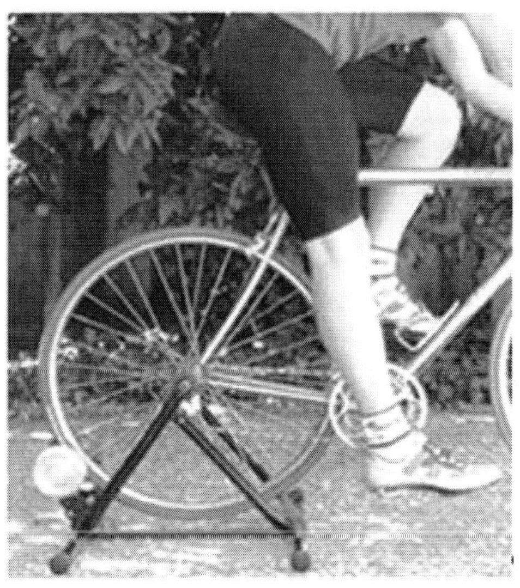

Don't raise the seat too much expecting to grow by an inch or even more at once. When the seat is raised too much, pedaling will be almost impossible and it's partly the reason why some complain of pain in the crotch.

On average, bones take 2 to 4 months to fully re-model so, the initial growth may happen after a short time but it will take about four months to gain approximately an inch in legs.

When you start growing, maintain the half inch increase and you will gradually continue adjusting as you grow.

Focus on the way the leg stretches.

Don't sprint cycle or pedal very fast, rather cycle casually making sure that the leg fully stretches out by attempting to reach the pedals with the instep or the arch of your foot.

You may get bored while performing this exercise so playing some music while subconsciously focusing on the way the legs stretch may help.

2 - 5 minutes of cycling every morning was enough to wear my legs out so I just did that every day though when starting out, 10 minutes or more a day will be ideal until the legs get used and you become fit as well.

The kind of bike to use

The other important factor is the type of bike to use. I suggest opting for a bike that will challenge you to mount.

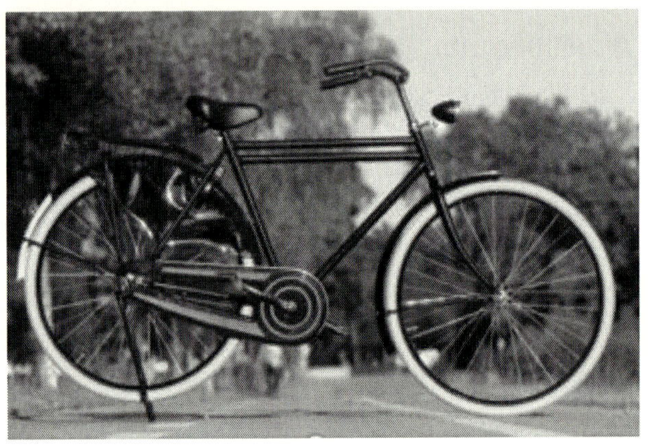

An example is the *Schwinn Hybrid Bike* or the *Dutch made roadmaster.* Don't use smaller bikes.

The bike also has to be stationary because it's quite challenging, if not impossible to efficiently pedal with a raised seat when the bike is in motion.

So, if you already have an outdoor bike, then just purchase a bike stand to make it stationed.

If you choose an indoor bike, opt for a bike with adjustable resistance levels. For instance, the Sunny *Health & Fitness SF-B1110* Indoor bike.

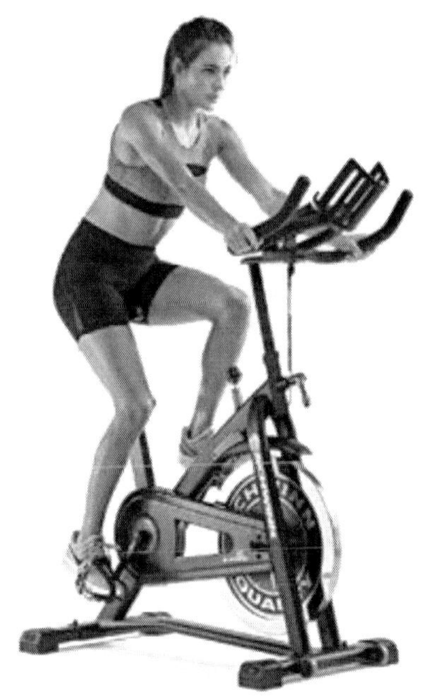

One of the challenges with most indoor bikes, is they come with short seat posts or stems making it impossible to adjust the stems.

The same may apply to some outdoor bikes. You may hire a welder to elongate your post or purchase an adjustable seat post.

When it comes to the resistance to use, let it just be moderate. Not too high and not too low. Just aim to mimic someone pedaling on level ground.

I suggest Medium resistance levels or levels around 10 or 11 depending on the brand of the bike.

The challenge

At first, it will seem impossible to cycle with the raised seat because you may feel like your bottom is getting ripped apart and it'll be quite sore for most people.

You will be tempted to quit during the first week or so, but I urge you to hang on.

After a week or two, you won't feel the pain anymore, and you'll get used.

PS: *Success stories with this technique using different cycling routines will be covered under the routines.*

B. Using Ankle weights.

This technique attempts to mimic the leg lengthening procedure.

The procedure is increasingly becoming a popular option for increasing leg length at any age for those who desire to have their legs lengthened though it is quite risky and prohibitively expensive.

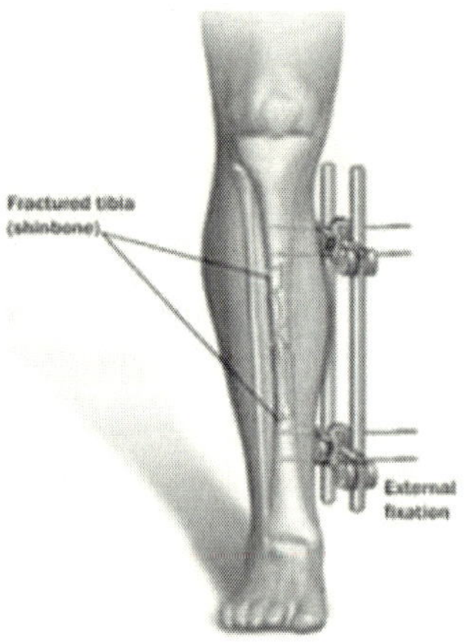

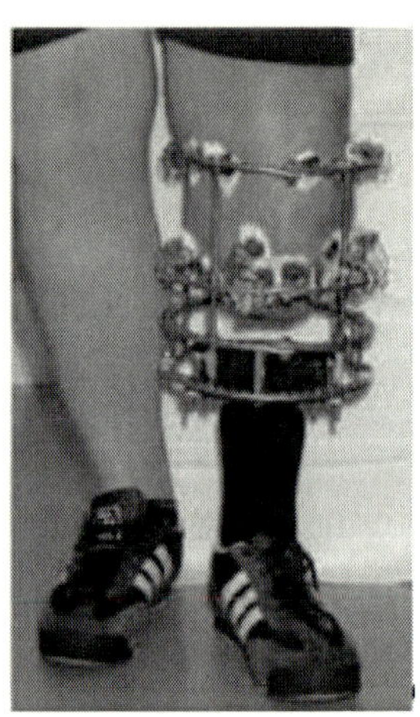

Leg lengthening surgery involves strategically breaking or cutting the shinbone and thigh bone into two then slowly separating the ends of the broken bone and allowing the separated parts of the bones to rejoin as the bone heals over a period of about 3 - 5 months.

The bone of course heals by manufacturing new bone between the created gaps.

Hence, to use ankle weights to lengthen legs, the idea is to create stress/ micro fractures first.

What is a stress or microfracture?

A stress/ micro fracture is a partially formed fracture as a result of increasing load or stress to a particular region of the bone.

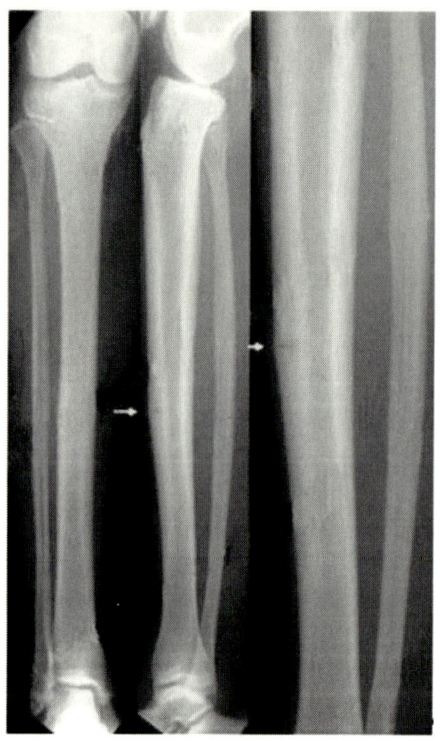

They form when you apply too much stress too often for the bone to recover or get used.

For instance, if you run too often at a high intensity on a hard surface for 5- 7 days a week without a break when the body isn't used to this kind of activity, stress fractures will form.

Micro fractures form gradually so, don't wait for clear signs of micro fractures to use ankle weights.

Every time you run or march with intensity, the bones weaken.

So, stretching them with ankle weights as they try to recover will be a good idea.

Hence, use ankle weights soon after running or marching with intensity. The earlier the better.

However, because of the way bones respond to stress, sometimes conditions like shin splints are mistaken to be micro fractures.

shin splints

Shin splints is pain and irritation you feel along the inner edge of shin bones especially the lower part of the shin bones after intense exercise especially on a hard surface.

The pain normally resolves after rest.

On the other hand, micro fracture pain is centered to the zone of the fracture and whenever you run or jump using the leg with the fracture, you feel discomfort until the fracture heals.

How to create microfractures.

The incidence of microfractures is highest among new military recruits or trainees and athletes due to the constant stamping of the feet during marching and running.

So, to create fractures, either spend plenty of time marching, jog or sprint on a hard surface every day for at least a week.

How do you know that you've created stress fractures?

1. Slight Pain in shin bone area after suddenly performing an exercise that requires marching or running at a very high intensity without giving leg bones ample time to rest and recover.

2. The Pain significantly subsides once you take a break from the exercise and this is the point when you should take a break from the activity that caused the microfracture but continue using the ankle weights.

3. The site of the micro or stress fracture may also be sensitive to touch.

4. When you jump with the leg under investigation and you feel any sharp pain in the shin bone area, then chances are high that the micro fracture is created.

How long do stress fractures take to heal?

With leg lengthening surgery, bone grows at a rate of approximately 1 mm per day or even more but it takes at least 6 -8 weeks for micro fractures to completely heal.

In other words, even when the fracture gap is completely sealed, it takes time for bone to completely solidify.

Note: More on how to use ankle weights covered under success stories.

C. Jumping.

I tried using jumping for some time but I wasn't successful.

However, a good number of folks say they successfully lengthen their legs by doing lots of jumps everyday so, I decided to include it here.

When the effects of jump training on bone hypertrophy *(growth)* were investigated in 3, 6, 12, 20- and 27-month-old female *Fischer rats,* the rats of all age groups jump trained 100 times a day for 5 days a week.

The fat-free dry weights *(weight of bone minus fat and water)* of the femur and the tibia were significantly greater in the jump-trained rats.

Jump training also significantly increased the length of the femur and the tibia as well as the diameter of the femur in both young and old rats.

The results of the study indicated that jump training was a more effective training mode than run training for bone hypertrophy and that the effects were not limited by age.

So, if you wish to try jumping, just go ahead. The Success story for jumping was also covered under success stories

THE TURNING POINT OF MY GROW TALLER CAMPAIGN

Before heading straight to the much-needed chapter, allow me to give you the climacteric of my grow taller campaign.

Chaos training.

This was the turning point when it came to my quest for height increase.

Before introducing chaos training to my exercise routine, I was only relying on sprints for G.H and after more than a year of exercising, I had managed to add 2- 3 inches of temporary height in the torso and about half an inch in legs.

Before I forget to mention, I started these exercises for height increase at 26 years and I was standing at 5'4". So, before chaos training, permanent height was 5'6.5". One inch was temporary.

With a much longer torso compared to legs, my body was definitely out of proportion, so I was desperate to do something about the length of my legs.

Many folks are concerned about growth plate's closure, and I was too, but at the same time, I was too desperate to give up especially after adding a few inches and being up beat that I could get more.

Hence, I decided to continue with my search for information then I came across *Adam Rainer* and *Vein Myllyrinne* stories.

These are some of the examples of individuals who experienced growth spurts throughout life even in their thirties because they were suffering from Acromegaly.

Acromegaly patients who are adults experience growth in feet fingers and skulls but these individuals experienced growth in all parts of their bodies until they died.

This yanked my attention and based on the knowledge I had regarding increasing growth hormones naturally in the body, on top of sprints which I was already doing, I added two techniques, both of which instigate growth hormone release.

One was weight lifting and the other was High Intensity Intermittent Exercising and this is what I call chaos training.

So, I hope now you understand why chaos training is so powerful.

More on how I used chaos training later. I didn't use fasting because I had quite a busy work schedule so eating was a must. *(Don't be concerned about acromegaly here unless of course you've a brain tumor. If too much G.H than is needed is released by the body, Somatostatin will come into play. This hormone was discussed in chapter 1.)*

Two to three weeks into chaos training, I started experiencing changes in my body structure.

First, my feet grew in length then I noticed my legs and feet became veiny.

At this point I didn't know what to expect. About a month or so later, I realized my fingers were a little longer.

I always had a little scar on my arm towards the elbow since my childhood years, but now it had moved upwards.

Then I took a closer look at my hands.

They were slightly longer. But this isn't what I was in for.

I wanted longer legs so, during all this time I continued with the cycling exercise hoping and praying.

But I hadn't noticed any significant increase in my shin bones.

Every once in a couple of days, I always felt spontaneous, piddling pains in my shin bones during my first month or two of cycling and sprinting before adding about a quarter of an inch in legs.

But now, with chaos training, the pains started becoming more regular.

One morning, when I was dressing up for work, the first pair of trousers I tried on wasn't fitting.

It was about a centimeter from the bottom of my feet. "What else could make the inseam shorter besides weight gain and leg length?" I wondered.

Excitedly I tried another pair of trousers confident that this was the moment I was waiting for. It didn't fit as well. It was an exuberant experience.

Before even measuring my height, this was the first proof that I had significantly grown in legs.

Not that I hadn't increased my height since I started exercising, but people will hardly notice that you're taller if your legs haven't significantly grown.

No one was telling me directly but I could hear voices in the background. People discussed my height because it was such a surprise considering my age.

Thus, all of the sudden I secretly became a topic of discussion at work and among family members.

I was beginning to tower over some of the hitherto taller workmates. But all I did was keep everything under wraps

CHAPTER 4

THE ROUTINE

Now that you have an insight on what it takes to increase height after puberty, it's time to share with you the exercise routine I successfully used plus the mistakes to avoid.

How age will influence your results.

1. ***12- 18 boys and Girls*** *(puberty years).*

Puberty is the stage in life when young boys and girls begin to transform into adults.

Teenagers become sexually mature and their bodies begin to transform into adult bodies.

This usually happens between ages 8 and 14 for girls and ages 9 and 16 for boys though in some cases it may end later for some teenagers.

If you're 18 years and under for most boys and girls, I don't advise you to use the routine as it is. Reason being that it involves chaos training to increase growth hormones. Chaos training includes weightlifting.

Excessive physical activity during childhood and adolescence may negatively affect body growth and adolescent development.

Excessive exercise is associated with delayed pubertal changes.

Sports that emphasize strict weight control in the setting of high-energy output are of particular concern.

Studies of male scholastic wrestlers have shown decreased linear growth during the sports season with catch-up growth during the post season.

Studies of elite female gymnasts and dancers have likewise demonstrated delayed growth and pubertal maturation during periods of intense training.

If you're still in puberty, your body is naturally undergoing the process of growth. Your body has the natural ability to release enough growth hormones to instigate growth.

You may however still utilize some of the exercises in this guide like cycling, ankle weights and the stretches

So, what should you do If you belong to this age group?

If you are in this age group, just center your efforts on other factors that facilitate body growth and human growth hormone production.

Some of these factors will be discussed further in the proceeding chapters.

They include but are not limited to;

A) Get involved in exercises or Sports that put stress on your legs.

Exercises, that require running, jumping or kicking out.

Such sports may include football, basketball, volleyball, handball and alike.

studies show that physical activity contributes a lot to muscle and bone development in physically

active children than in those who aren't physically active.

B) Avoid early sex not masturbation.

I receive a couple of emails from adolescent boys wondering if masturbation is responsible for their stunted growth.

According to rcscarch conductcd by John Morris a doctoral student in psychology and his team on 40-day old hamsters; *(which they say are equivalent to old teenagers in human terms)* early sex can affect the immune system and delay the onset of puberty and growth, as well as having 'lasting effects on the body and mood' which continue into adulthood.

This is because the teen body interprets sex as a "stressor," sending the immune system into

behind conditions such as IBS *(Irritable Bowel Syndrome)* which can delay the onset of puberty and affect growth because sufferers miss out on crucial nutrients.

C) Growth hormone therapy

In 2003, the *Food Drug Administration* of the United states approved the treatment of short stature with recombinant human growth hormone and such therapy has proven to be effective in increasing height velocity and increasing chances of the child reaching adult height.

That's what the Argentine endocrinologist *Diego Schwarzstein* did for the now famous footballer Lionel Messi in 1998 when diagnosed with a partial growth hormone deficiency.

In a study that aimed to investigate the efficacy of recombinant growth hormones in increasing height velocity among pre pubertal south Korean children with short stature, it was found that those who were treated with 0.067 mg per kg weight of recombinant growth hormones for 6 months grew more rapidly after 6 months.

D) Improve your nutrition.

If you're still in puberty or yet to enter puberty, Emphasis should be on the following foods;

i) Milk at least 500mls low fat every day.

ii) Zinc rich foods. Mainly oysters, crabs and beef. If you for some reason you can't consume these foods, Supplement with 30 – 40 milligrams every day. The body doesn't require more than 50mgs every day.

iii) At least 0.8g of protein per kg weight every day. With animal meats and products like eggs and milk, you can easily reach the target.

If you're vegetarian, quinoa and soy beans will do.

iv) Plenty of tinned fish for vitamin D or if you can access the sun, the better.

v) Take at least 2 liters of water every day

E) Sleep, sleep and sleep.

Like already mentioned, everything related to growth of bone takes place when you're sleeping. So, capitalize on the time when the body is rapidly growing by having plenty of sleep.

F) Delay growth plates closure.

According to studies, there are a couple of supplements and drugs you can use to delay the closure of your growth plates if you are still in puberty.

Such medicines and supplements include Resveratrol, Tamoxifen and aromatase inhibitors like Arimidex and Letrozole.

2. 20 - 26 years

Most success declarations come from this age group so if you belong to this age group; you have higher chances of growing after puberty.

3. 27 years and above

If you belong to this age group, you may face a number of challenges that may prevent or impede your success. Since I started at 26, I encountered some of these challenges but don't despair; there's still hope.

I say this because I once received an email from a 37-year-old who claimed he added 3cm in legs with ankle weights, but he never reverted when I asked what exactly he did.

He only shared pictures; then another email from a 38-year-old who added 2.5 inches in torso between 38 and 40years.

Since for most people this is the busiest time of their life, the principle challenge faced by folks 27 years and over is inconsistency.

If you don't have the time to focus on the routine, you'll have limited chances to make it.

I quit my day job to focus on the routine just because I realized that during my leave, I grew more rapidly.

Then after quitting my job, I started growing consistently.

I don't advise you to do the same, but just sharing my personal experience.

4. The Athletes

The other category that faces challenges with the routine is the athletes.

Most athletes have regular training sessions so incorporating the grow taller routine with the training routine becomes a big challenge.

First, to be successful with the routine, you need plenty of rest.

If you're an athlete and you train twice or three times a week, then I suggest you do all the chaos training exercises on the same day.

The stretches, cycling and ankle weights routines may be done any day regardless of training routine

The other challenge is that the athlete body is used to physical activity so muscles are almost fully stretched.

Third, when it comes to increasing growth hormones release, shocking the body with chaos training or sprints to release G.H will be a challenge since most athletes do plenty of sprints and some lift weights on a daily basis.

So, the athletes need to exercise with a lot of intensity to reach the lactate thresh hold with chaos training.

Finally, when it comes to creating microfractures, with time the bones adapt to the incoming stress whenever an athlete runs or jumps.

Bones adapt by becoming thicker thus, creating microfractures in an athlete's leg bones will be a bear.

Hence, most athletes have to either work hard or be persistent to create microfractures.

What is needed?

This routine will mainly focus on upper body and lower body that is; the most effective torso lengthening stretches including the neck and chest stretches as well as abdominal workouts.

For the lower body, emphasis is on lengthening the shin bones with either cycling with raised saddle, or using ankle weights.

Jumping will only be discussed under success stories because I never spent much time on jumps.

If your budget is tight, this routine can be performed in the comfort of your home besides sprints which will require a pitch or clearing of approximately half a football pitch.

You can as well utilize the stairs and run on them as a substitute for sprints provided, they are long enough.

Otherwise, the following equipment may be required;

1. An indoor cycling bike.

2. Alternatively, use an outdoor bicycle like a hybrid bike.

3. A bicycle stand to make the outdoor bike stationary.

4. Hanging bar.

5. Dumbbells

6. Ankle Weights

7. Inflatable cushion or Spine Stretching Therapeutic Device.

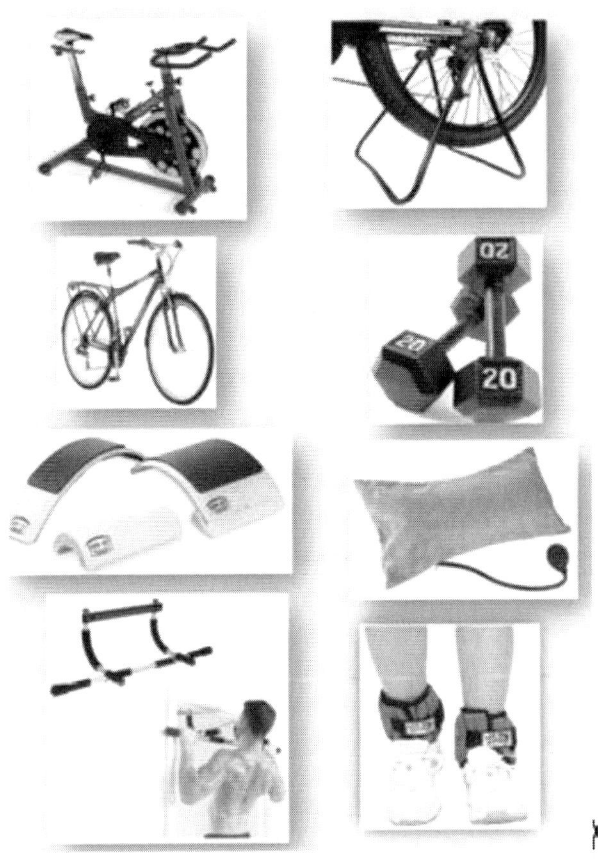
20
20
20

EXERCISES THAT WILL BE PERFORMED IN THIS ROUTINE IN DETAIL

First, there is potential to grow in four areas of your body and all these areas have specific exercises that target them.

These areas include;

1. The neck

2. The chest

3. The Abdominal area or back bone

4. The shin bones

.1. The neck

Stand still or erect with your head straight.

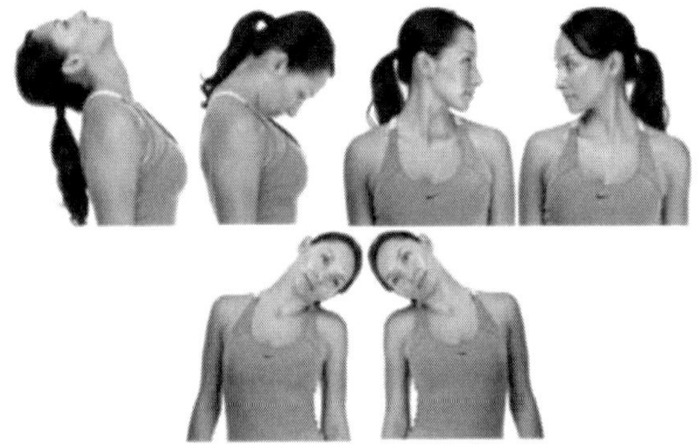

Then Stretch your neck towards the left by tilting your head over to the left shoulder for 5 to 10 seconds and do the same by stretching your neck towards the right shoulder for 5 to 10 seconds.

Next, fall your head to the back and be able to look at the ceiling for 5 to 10 seconds and do the same with your head facing the floor.

After the entire workout, roll your head around. Repeat the entire work out 2-3 times.

I suggest you do this every morning together with the chest stretches which will be discussed below or just before doing the other stretches otherwise it's easy to abandon or forget about the neck and chest stretches.

2. *The chest stretch.*

Perform this exercise by firmly holding the position as indicated in the picture for at least 10 seconds and perform this exercise just after and every time you stretch your neck to effectively stretch the thoracic spine.

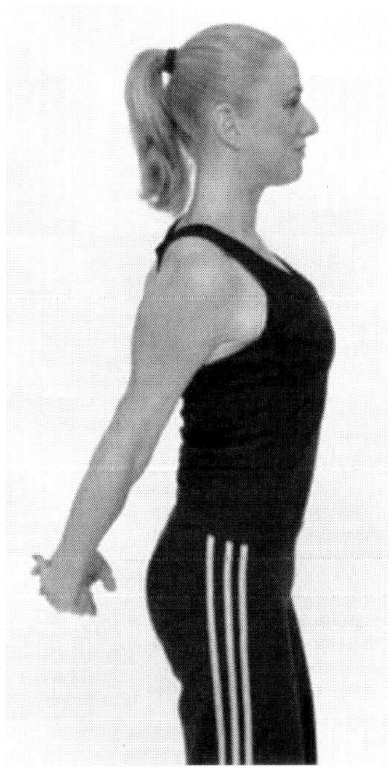

3. *The Abdominal area or trunk.*

Four stretching exercises, a back-stretching device or inflatable cushion and two abdominal workouts are very effective.

A. The Stretches

Hanging

This is the most effective and important of all the stretches. So, if you have nowhere to hang, at least improvise. Any bar high enough to hang with the feet off the floor will do.

Hang to the count of at least 30seconds every morning and evening just before going to bed every day as a must.

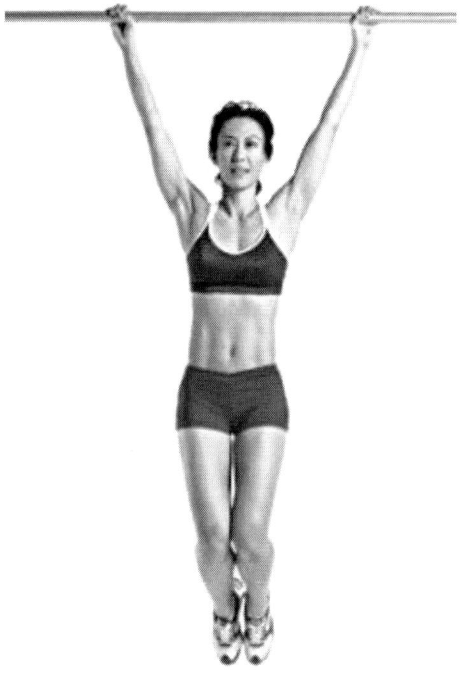

In the beginning, you may struggle to make 30 seconds but with time, it will be much easier and you will be able to hang on even longer.

Dry swimming

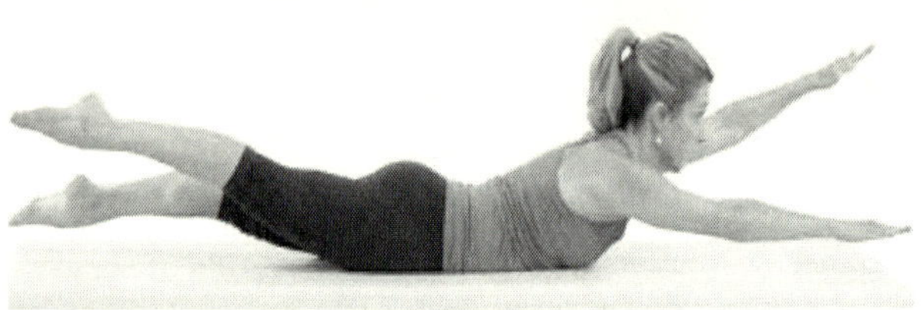

Lie prone on the floor, then Raise your left hand diagonally off the ground in sync with your right leg as illustrated above and hold a position for 5 to 10 seconds.

Relax for a couple of seconds before switching to the left leg and right hand.

Do 1 to 3 repetitions before relaxing the back bone by performing the cat stretch.

Cat stretch

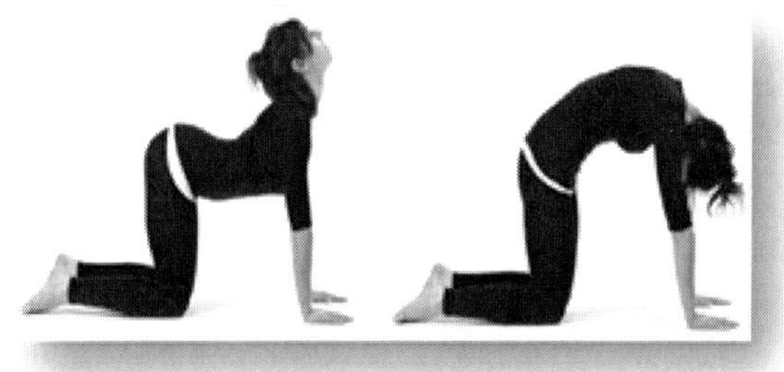

Get on all fours with your arms locked out.

Inhale as you flex your spine down and bring your head up. Exhale as you bring your spine up into an arched position while bringing your head down. Hold positions for 5 - 10 seconds.

Cobra Stretch

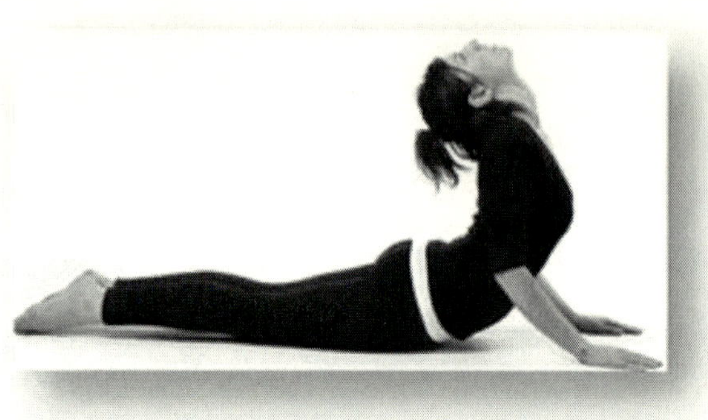

Be prone on the floor with your hands positioned directly under your shoulders and fingers facing forward. Legs should be straight and toes pointed.

Upward Phase: Gently inhale.

Engage your abdominal/core muscles to support the spine. Press your hips into the mat or floor.

Lengthen the torso and curl your chest away from the ground while keeping your hips stable. Keep the shoulders rolling down and back. Hold this position for 15 - 30 seconds.

Downward Phase: Gently lower your upper body back to the mat or floor, lengthening the spine as you descend.

Using the back arcing or spine stretching device and Inflatable cushion.

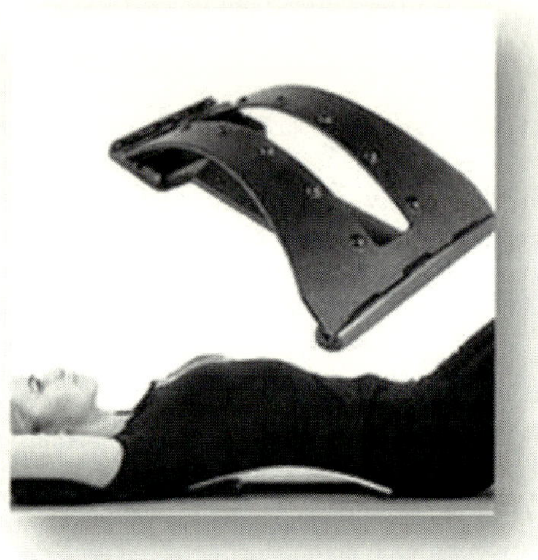

These come in different shapes, types and sizes but they are relatively cheap ranging from $15.

Either use this device or the inflatable cushion everyday especially if you have nowhere to hang but hanging is very important.

Place the inflatable cushion or device at the arc of your spine or the lower back area.

The hanging exercise, back arcing or inflatable cushion are very important for rehydrating the spinal discs and undo the impact of prolonged sitting especially with a poor posture.

So, all the three help to increase and maintain torso height.

A lot of torso height is lost with poor sitting posture.

If you can't secure an inflatable cushion in the meantime though, you may improvise by creating your own cushion and lic supinc on it.

This is very important especially in advanced stage when the muscles are fully stretched, and the body is accustomed to all the stretches.

That is; at the time when you don't feel the stretching impact any more.

Lie on the inflatable cushion or back arc for at least 10 minutes. You can do this while watching TV or engaging in any other activity like meditating as time passes.

At the end of the day, you will have a healthy spine, your back will thank you and you will be a couple of millimeters if not centimeters taller in the torso.

B. Abdominal / core Exercises

Two abdominal workouts were effective during the routine.

Sit ups

These are very effective when done immediately after the stretches. They will help you get a stronger core and stabilize torso height.

Begin by lying supine to the floor, with the arms across the chest or behind the head and knees bent and then elevate both the upper and lower vertebrae from the floor until the entire upper body is not touching the ground.

Do 5 to 10 reps in the beginning then do as many as you can when you get used.

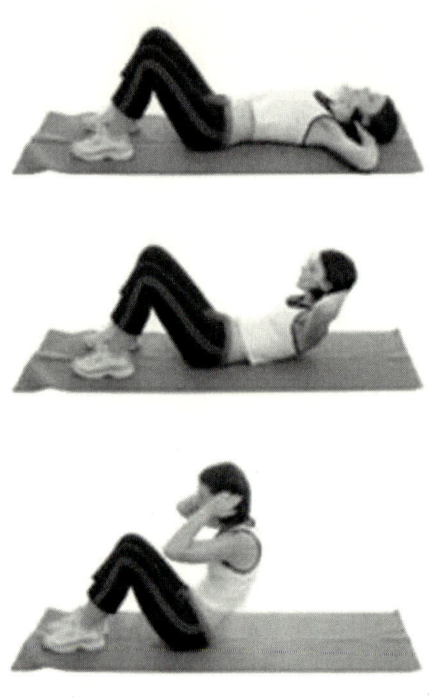

Push ups

These will be part of chaos training but you can do them after sit-ups.

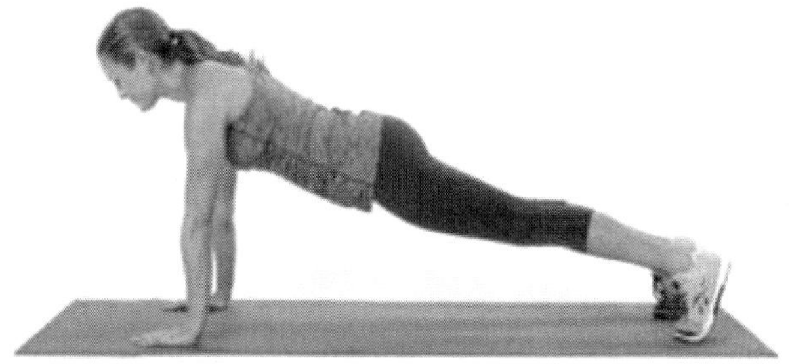

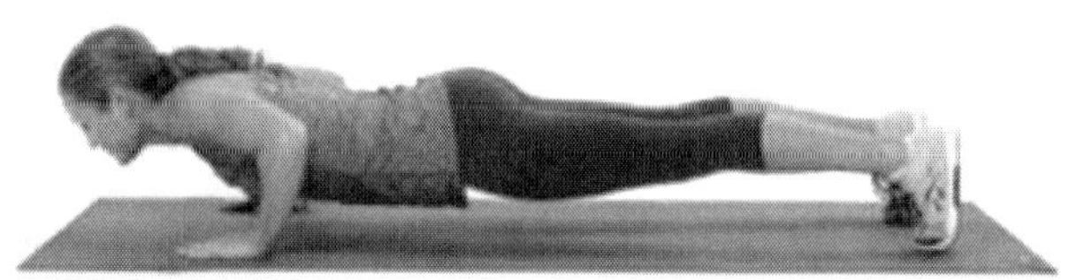

4. LENGTHENING THE SHIN BONES

There are many exercises that will lengthen shin bones but I will focus on four effective ones.

The effective exercises include;

a. Cycling with raised saddle

b. Sprinting

c. Chaos training.

d. Using Ankle weights

A. Cycling with raised saddle

Enough has already been said about this in chapter 3.

B. Sprinting.

This exercise should also be performed when doing the stretches for G.H

Many ask if they should do plenty of sprints for more G.H. But like earlier mentioned, metabolic responses are greatest after the 30 second sprint and more G.H remains elevated after sprinting for 30 seconds than after sprinting for 60 minutes.

It's a case of diminishing returns. With more sprints, the body gets used and less G.H is released.

Hence, perform this exercise by covering a distance of 40 to 60 yards.

1- 3 sessions depending on your fitness levels.

A session, in this case, is sprinting 40-60 yards four times.

At the time I started the exercises, I wasn't fit at all, so one session was enough in my case. ***(That is; sprint 40-60 yards going, and 40-60 yards coming back at a top speed. That is two times.)***

I did one session, but if you are an athlete or feel fit enough and you have the time then you may take a break for 5 or so minutes and do the second session.

If you have a problem determining the number of yards, then just sprint at top speed going until you feel too exhausted to carry on and do the same coming back and repeat.

Do these sprints nonstop four times (one session) for about 30 seconds to 1 minute to raise the anaerobic (lactate) threshold.

The entire session doesn't last more than 2 minutes.

Note: That's exactly what I did partly because it was enough to wear me out and I didn't have plenty of time for the exercises.

C. Chaos training *(High-Intensity Intermittent Training or Exercises)*

As explained earlier, short bursts of high-intensity (or max-intensity) exercises, should be followed by a brief low-intensity activity, repeatedly, until too exhausted to continue typically within 30 minutes.

This may include a set of 3- 5 strength training exercises performed intermittently with the aim of exhausting the muscles quickly so that enough growth hormone is released.

Weight lifting exercises are part of the set of exercises simply because weight lifting is one of the exercises that can trigger growth hormone release.

So, lifting weights intermittently will double the potential to trigger G.H release since H.I.I.T/E autonomously sparks G.H release.

I will explain this again;

When muscle tissue contracts intensely for an extended period, the blood circulation system starts to lose ground in the circulation of fresh air necessary for energy release.

In these circumstances, the breakdown of sugar is changed to lactic acid.

As the lactate is created in the muscle tissue, it oozes out into the bloodstream and is distributed around our bodies.

If this situation continues, our body performance reduces, and the muscle tissue wears out very quickly. This point is often calculated as the lactate limit/ threshold.

The point when the muscle is fatigued to the point of almost failing to move voluntarily.

Like earlier explained, an increase in blood lactic acid levels is a significant trigger of human growth hormone (H.G.H) release.

Four exercises I included in this set of exercises to exhaust as many muscles that is;

Sprinting

Sprints alone trigger G.H release, but Weight lifting releases more G.H.

They are part of the chaos training set of exercises to involve as many muscle groups as possible which renders chaos training more complete.

Followed by push-ups

Then two Weight lifting exercises which are;

Shoulder fly

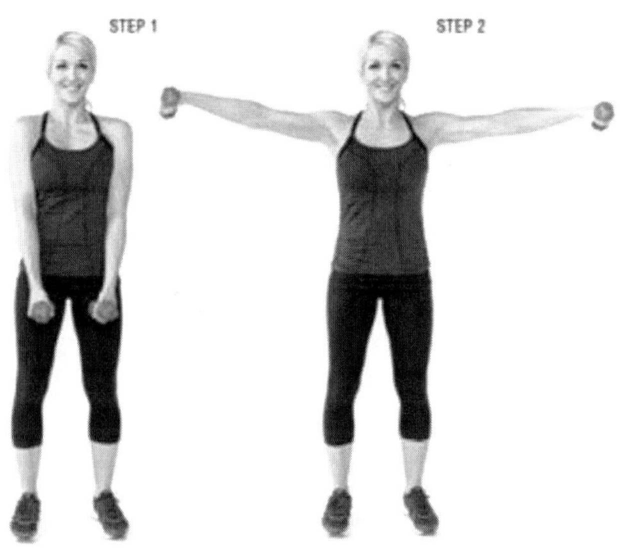

Stand with hands holding down weights. Make sure you use lifts heavy just enough depending on your strength.

Not too heavy and not too light. 2- 10kgs will do for most people.

Use slightly lighter weights for your weaker hand.

Then move the hands upwards gently while fully stretched out and when you reach the shoulder level, gently lower them.

Do up to 5 to 10 repetitions depending on your level of strength or simply do repetitions to the point where you can't push it any further then take a breather for 5 or so seconds before switching to the next work out.

Chest Fly

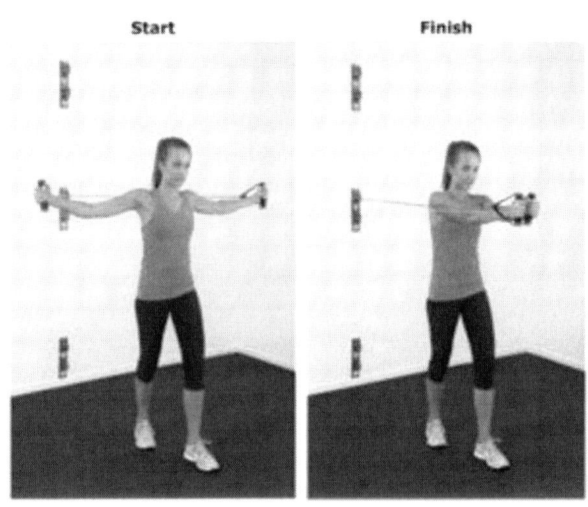

You don't necessarily need resistance bands to execute this workout. Dumbbells are enough.

Stretch the hands out gently and move them back until they meet.

Do five to ten repetitions. The pectorals and triceps, as well as forearms, will be worked out with this exercise.

More on when to do chaos training and how will be discussed later under the routine.

SYNOPSIS OF MY SUCCESSFUL ROUTINE IN DETAIL

During the first 1 to 3 *Months (Beginner's stage)*

It's during the first month that intensity may be of benefit, but this intensity will only apply to stretching exercises.

You will need to intensely stretch, to loosen the muscles as quick as Possible.

If you are targeting torso lengthening

At the time I started I was working part time so I had plenty of time for the workouts.

The freer you are, the better and faster you may notice results.

Every day in the morning when you wake up, do the chest and neck stretches.

These should be done first thing in the morning as your early morning stretches.

Then do the hanging exercise. Hang for at least thirty seconds 2 to 3 repetitions.

Then do the cobra stretch with 2 to 3 repetitions, then dry swim two to three times.

Finally, cat stretch once. Repeat if you wish since this isn't as strenuous as other stretches.

Immediately after the stretches, do abdominal workouts. I suggest 5-10 sit-ups or even more if you wish.

Sit-ups may be done once a day.

These strengthen your core muscles and help to stabilize any gains you may achieve in the torso.

Walk during the day, whenever you get the opportunity.

Repeat the series of the stretching exercises during the day if you wish and do the same at night before bed.

Otherwise, twice a day morning and night is enough.

Later in the evening, go for the sprint session. Every day, continue the entire stretching routine morning and evening.

Please remember that stretching alone will not make you taller.

You will require growth hormones to facilitate any form of growth. Let it be muscles, cartilage or bones. That's why you will need the sprints during the first one to three months.

From the day you do the first sprint session, skip two days before the second session.

If your first sprint session is on Monday, skip 2 days before the second on Thursday, and the third on Sunday and that will be three times of sprinting a week.

However, if you begin on Tuesday, then you may sprint twice a week if you maintain the two-day gap between sprint sessions.

That means, if you are just beginning, you will be sprinting 2-3 times a week but no chaos training particularly weight lifting at this stage.

Endeavour to perform the sprinting exercise on a hard surface rather than a treadmill for optimal results.

In the beginning, you will need to perform the torso stretches every day, and your torso may keep growing.

Initially, it will be slow progress but as time passes by with better nutrition and more growth hormones released in the body, the torso will grow more rapidly.

Don't fret, if these workouts are a bit strenuous in the beginning.

You may consider giving up, but the strain will be due to lack of fitness thus your muscles won't stretch without you feeling some strain.

After a couple of days of stretching, your muscles will loosen, you will feel comfortable, and everything will simply be a piece of cake.

There are so many stretching exercises that target the backbone, but it will be better to concentrate a few that you can perform every day for the first month for an efficient stretching routine.

Though when starting out you will feel the urge to try out every exercise you come across, that's fine.

Our bodies are different thus you may come across more effective stretches for your body than the above-listed exercises.

Otherwise, if you fail to grow, then try to focus on the above-recommended exercises to see if there will be a positive effect.

However, after one to three months, the strain felt while performing these exercises will reduce and if this is the case, then eliminate all other exercises and do only hanging, and sit-ups or use the back-arcing device/ inflatable cushion and sit ups.

Otherwise, time comes when your torso can grow no more no matter the stretching exercise.

Most importantly, Watch your sitting posture very closely.

It's the principle culprit for losing your torso height since most of us spend most of the time seated.

After one to three months, you may be noticing a slight difference in your torso height unless something wasn't done right.

Otherwise, some report positive results after as early as two weeks.

How to know that you are on the right track with torso lengthening after following the routine strictly;

First, your upper body will begin to loosen and look frail because the hitherto compact muscles are now stretched.

Your neck will also slacken and become weaker. This shouldn't bother you, since over time, these muscles will regroup with the aid of a high protein diet and they will be compact with a new length.

You will also realize that the hitherto fitting tops (shirt or blouse) will not be fitting you anymore and you will need to keep purchasing new attire more often because your upper body will be blossoming.

Shin Bone lengthening if you are starting out.

Since I used cycling, I will only focus on cycling for now.

Please note that I independently tried other leg lengthening exercises like kicking out, jumping rope and ankle weights as I was looking for a stationary bike but in vain.

These exercises may have prepared my body because after securing the bike, I noticed results just after two to three weeks.

You may choose to do the cycling routine in the morning or evening but for at least 10 minutes if you are just starting out.

Therefore, for shin bone lengthening, you will only focus on cycling and sprints during the first 1 - 3 months. Sprints will be used as a trigger for G.H release.

Thus, sprints were central throughout my routine.

Feel free to use other methods for increasing G.H like fasting but don't overdo it.

If you choose to fast, I suggest you fast on the days you sprint.

If you wish to use ankle weights, I will share *Jeff* and *Evan's* stories later. And you may follow their ankle weights routines.

If you wish to try jumping, *Jieyangcen* shared his success routine with jumping under success stories. So, back to the cycling routine, just pedal with raised saddle every day and sprint three times a week.

Below is how bone formation and growth take place after applying stress on legs.

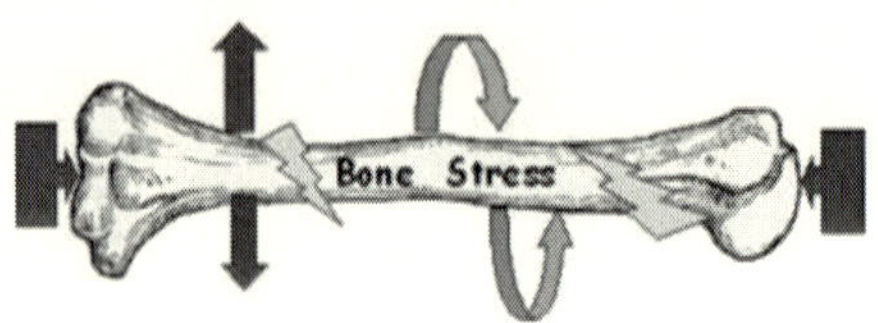

1) Compression (pressing together)
2) Tension (pulling apart)
3) Torsion (Twisting)
4) Shear (tearing across)

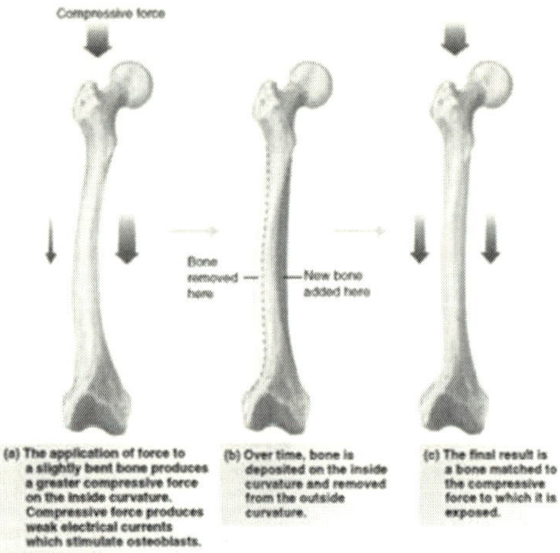

(a) The application of force to a slightly bent bone produces a greater compressive force on the inside curvature. Compressive force produces weak electrical currents which stimulate osteoblasts.

(b) Over time, bone is deposited on the inside curvature and removed from the outside curvature.

(c) The final result is a bone matched to the compressive force to which it is exposed.

In brief, below is the complete beginner level routine.

When you wake up, begin with the stretches that is; Chest and neck stretch, hanging, cobra, dry swimming and cat stretch. Then do the sit ups.

After the sit ups, pedal with a raised seat for 5- 10 minutes but if you have time, feel free to pedal for longer.

The most important thing is doing this everyday not time spent pedaling.

You may repeat the stretches during the day, before going for the sprints in the evening.

Then repeat the stretches before bedtime.

Follow the same routine every day besides the sprints which you will have to do once every two days.

I will throw more light later on why you shouldn't sprint every day.

One question I'm always asked is "can you do both the torso and shin bone routine at once?" The answer is yes.

I just summarized that above.

So that's it.

A very easy to follow yet effective beginner stage routine. It is easy but some mistakes which I explained later under the mistakes to avoid will be the biggest stumbling block.

Some of you access this book when you've done the stretches before.

If you've been stretching for some time, the advanced stage routine is discussed below.

***Advanced stage.** (If you've been doing the routine for some time and you are a bit flexible)*

This is when chaos training will be introduced to the routine.

The chaos training routine.

Sprinting is part of the chaos training exercises.

Therefore, sprint on the day you lift weights and do this twice a week.

Thus, chaos training may include all the following exercises on the same day.

First, sprint. If the field or area where you sprint is distant, no need to bother. The other set of exercises may be done separately.

Therefore, sprint not necessarily the time you do the rest of chaos training exercises.

Even hours earlier.

Then do 10 to 20 pushups depending on the amount that wears you out.

Followed by the chest fly 10 to 20 reps depending on the reps that exhaust your arms.

Then again, 10 to 20 push ups before finally performing the shoulder fly 10 - 20 reps.

Remember to maintain a rest period of about 15 - 30 seconds in between the exercises reason being that if you rest for long, the muscles will be allowed to recover before you have worked them hard enough and it will require you more time to exhaust them to that point when they can't voluntarily move.

The entire work out may be done consecutively within 5-10 minutes, but it will be useful in helping the body release more growth hormones.

The point here is to work out the muscles quickly to the point when they can't voluntarily move.

For efficient results, first, have your protein-rich dinner before these exercises.

By the time you finish the last exercise, you will be completely worn out. Take a quick shower before going to bed.

Make sure you sleep for at last 8 hours especially on the day you do chaos training exercises otherwise your body may fail to fully recover from this chaotic exercising and you may feel lethargic throughout the next day.

It's essential to do chaos training exercises late in the evening because of the following reasons;

i) After performing these exercises, you will feel so exhausted a recipe for slow wave sleep (very deep sleep). Remember, it's during slow wave sleep that most G.H is released.

ii) Sleep researchers have predicted that; total sleep time, and slow wave sleep would be higher in physically fit individuals than those who are unfit and higher on nights following exercise.

iii) If you are the type who goes to bed then struggle to get sleep, on the days you perform these exercises, sleep will not be a problem.

In fact, normally when you exercise, you fall asleep faster, have a deeper sleep, wake up less often, and feel less tired during the day.

This prediction is based on the "compensatory" position, which suggests that "draining" daytime activity (like exercise) would most likely result in a compensatory increase in the need for night time sleep, thereby facilitating recuperative, restorative and energy conservation processes.

iv) Our bodies recover more efficiently when sleeping than when we are awake.

So, your body may stay fatigued if you do these exercises in the morning or during the day.

Combine the need to recover your muscles, slow wave sleep, and the fact that most G.H is released at night all of which make late evening the best time for chaos training.

Important to note;

Don't expect your body to initiate another growth spurt long after puberty without conditioning or giving it preparation and this is where many get it wrong.

So, make sure during the first 1-3 months, you do sprints alone before introducing chaos training.

This will allow you to understand your body better and know what works for your body. If your body doesn't grow during the first 1 to 3 months, you may be able to identify your mistakes.

If you successfully notice results even before two months when performing only sprints for G.H, then you are on the right track and at this point, you may introduce the chaos exercises for more growth hormones to be released in the body and this will be the beginning of a new growth spurt.

The summary of advanced stage routine.

Starting day, say Wednesday.

By this time, your body will be used to the stretches so, stretch your chest and neck before Hanging for 30 seconds first thing in the morning.

If you've nowhere to hang, employ the back-arcing device or inflatable cushion for 10 minutes or use both hanging and inflatable cushion.

Then do 10 or so sit-ups.

That's all with the torso routine thus, immediately jump onto your stationary bike.

Pedal for about 2-5 minutes casually. Make sure you do not rush this.

Within 10 to 15 minutes you will be through with the entire routine.

Assuming you work, study or have a busy daytime, when you come back from work in the evening, take dinner between 7 PM -8 PM by the time you do the sprints at about 9, insulin levels will be much lower in the blood.

The point is to do chaos training hours after eating not to suppress G.H levels in the blood.

Remember, insulin levels spike especially immediately after eating carbohydrates and insulin suppresses growth hormone release.

So, take more amino acid-rich proteins and minimal carbohydrates especially on the day you do chaos training.

Begin with the sprints later in the evening.

Many face the challenge of finding enough clearing for the sprints and end up using treadmills.

I suggest you use walkways to your home instead. Any clear distance as long as 15- 20 m may do.

After the sprints, use your dumbbells to do chaos training. Remember, it's still Wednesday the starting day.

Every day, follow the morning stretching routine and let it be part of your life like brushing your teeth. Trust me, the morning stretches are awesome.

Four days after Wednesday, that is Sunday, do chaos training again.

I realized that when I started taking 4 to 5 days without chaos training because of unavoidable circumstances; I grew more rapidly than when I took 1 – 3 days between chaos training.

Thus, the body needs ample time to recover. And doing it more often makes the body more accustomed to the chaos training then less G.H will be released.

The same explains why there should be a 48-hour time lag between the sprints in the beginning. If you follow the 4 to 5-day rest period, you will also realize that you will do chaos training once a week during some weeks.

That's it for the advanced stage routine. It looks simple, but it's efficient. Remember to Just avoid the mistakes.

If you are targeting growth in shin bones, take note of this;

With shin bone lengthening, you need to know that the bone can't grow without enough growth hormones in the body.

If you 're targeting growth in the shin bones, all your efforts should be centered on doing whatever it takes to stimulate the Pituitary gland so it releases enough G.H for your body to grow because without enough growth hormones, whatever you do will be a waste of time.

For starters, sprints alone will be chaotic enough. But later you will need to introduce chaos training Exercises.

At least 8 hours of quality sleep on a daily basis will also be a must.

Now when it comes to milk, I have to place a disclaimer. Milk is very good, but don't take too much of it. I used to take two glasses every day which is about 500mls to get faster results.

Whole milk contains lots of sugars which may lead to Weight gain so take it in limited quantities. And too much insulin like growth factor 1 in adults which is contained in milk is linked to cancer.

It’s not advised to take more than three glasses a day. But low-fat milk is relatively safe.

On the other hand, the Insulin-like growth factor 1 hormone contained in milk is very important for cell division and body growth.

So, if taking milk doesn't cause any health concerns for you, then you should have 1 to 2 glasses every day.

Then also, have enough amino acids rich Proteins mainly egg whites, beef, fish, and poultry like chicken and turkey. These animal proteins coupled with milk will play a significant role.

Enough was said about them under nutrition.

Missing out on any of the above essential factors may be enough to fail you in achieving your goal.

That is; sleep, G.H, nutrition, consistency, and how you do the exercises.

Some of this will be discussed under the mistakes to avoid.

How to know that you are on the right track with shin bone lengthening;

since I used cycling, I will share my experience with cycling.

First, there will be spontaneous, fleeting and piddling pains both in the shin bone and around the knee cap during any time of the day.

These pains will not last more than 5 to 10 minutes then they will disappear. They may resurface once or twice during the same day but may sparingly resurface during the next day.

A week or two later, you will notice the knee cap bones slightly widened and or conspicuous.

Then these bones thicken as time passes by and the thickness may account for the first quarter to half an inch gain in the legs. With time, the shin bones also begin to lengthen.

Your feet will also be able to reach the pedals even when the seat is raised before increasing it to the next level. That's if you slightly increased the seat post.

My feet grew slightly before my shin bones but this will not always signal shin bone growth.

All other factors constant, like weight gain, the most obvious sign of leg growth will be the difference in your trouser inseam length.

A few Pointers when following this exercise routine.

When performing these stretches, you'll feel back pain every once in a while. Either perform a dry swim lie on an inflatable cushion or hang to get some relief.

The pain may be the result of back bones relocating to their hitherto positions before the stretches.

If your objective is to solely add a couple of inches to your height, then a few changes will have to be effected in your daily activity routine and that means you'll need to make height increase a priority.

If it means clearing sometime and give these grow taller exercises a priority, then do that.

This routine will be perfect if you are desperate enough to give it 100% dedication. Many folks over 5'6" may not gain that much in height merely because they lack the zeal to stick to the routine for long.

You need to know that height gained after puberty through stretching the torso is never permanent unless either the spinal discs are rehydrated or enough growth hormone is released in the body to facilitate cartilage, muscle and or bone growth including backbones to support your height gain.

So, you have to continue hanging and or using the inflatable cushion to rehydrate the discs.

Abdominal workouts may also stabilize the gains.

"MOST IMPORTANT TO NOTE; IS THAT

THE BODY NEEDS MORE RECOVERY

THAN INTENSITY"

CHAPTER 5

LEG LENGTHENING WITH EXERCISES SUCCESS STORIES

A. Leg lengthening with cycling success stories

Note: *The following success stories were picked from a cycling forum as they were without any editing. They were from real people and they're quitc crcdiblc.*

1) posted by: Leo

When I was 23 years old, I used to cycle to college which was about 10 miles away- s there and back is 20 miles in total. I read somewhere about increasing saddle height

so, your legs are stretched when you cycle - so it gives a slight pull on the legs. It's bloody sore to start off with but you get used to it after a week.

I done this every day for 4 months (along with plenty of protein drinks) and increased the length of my legs by over 2.5 inches - increasing saddle height 1/4 inch every few weeks.

I honestly believe that any one regardless of age can achieve this and more - the legs are literally forced to grow to accommodate all that pulling and stretching.

But I never see anyone else singing the

praises of cycling to increase height - am I the only one?

2) posted by: Anonymous

"Cycling for height"July 10 2002 at 5:31 AM

Anonymous: *Well, I don't know if this is true but I know I increased the length of my legs a few years ago by doing the cycling exercise whereby you have to make sure your legs are fully stretched.*

I used to cycle 15 miles a day and the growth was really rapid - and I was 27 years old. I'm surprised this sort of thing isn't featured more on this forum as it really works.

Ann's question for anonymous: *Was the height you gained in your legs permanent? How much did you gain? So simply cycling should* *help or are there stretches/exercises for the legs specifically that would get the same results?*

Anonymous' response: *Yes, it was permanent.*

I just made sure I cycled every day and I ate a healthy diet supplemented with protein powder.

I also got at least 8 hours sleep a night. I just can't see why all you people find it so hard to increase your height - it's easy.

If you put the effort in and stay healthy then the growth will come.

An interesting point is that when I cycled for just 6 to 7 miles a day not much happened but when I cycled 15 miles every day then I really noticed the increase. I used to increase the saddle height 1/4 almost every 2 weeks.

Anonymous' other post: *"It was me who posted that"*

Well I'm glad some people took some notice of my post –I haven't visited this site for a while because nobody seemed interested in this method of height increase. Like I said, to notice the effect… 5, 6, 7 miles isn't enough.

You must do at least 15 miles of hard cycling and make sure that your legs and feet are stretching every time.

If you're doing it properly – and eating correctly – it should only take a couple of weeks to gain ¼ inch.

Obviously, the younger you are the better the results you are going to get but you can still get good results no matter how old you are.

This is the best method of height increase I know and more people should put the effort in and at least give it a try.

You have to do a lot of miles almost every day.

3) posted by BG :

I grew an inch from cycling. I joined a serious cycling club and did about 40 kms a week.

I have grown from under 5'11 to 6'0, my goal is 6'1.

I was very pleased with this as I tried 100 other methods including hanging, stretching and basketball, and I never grew a cm.

1 km = 0.621 mile... 40 km = 24.8 miles

4) posted by: 5ft8guy:

"Really?"

September 11, 2003, 1:10 AM

For real? you grew by raising the saddle? I used to ride my bike to work and I liked to make my saddle height really high. I was like 5'4.5 or 5'5

when I was 15 and I became 5'8 when I turned 16. then I got my driver's license and never bike to work again and i never grew anymore.

Let me know if you kept on growing by raising the saddle, I wanna know if it really helps!

keep this thread updated.

B. LEG LENGTHENING WITH ANKLE WEIGHTS SUCCESS STORIES

How Vulcrum* (Jeff) *grew 2.5 inches in the legs within 5 months.

Nickname: *Vulcrum- Real name is Jeff.*

Age : *15 years old.*

Sex : Male

Ethnicity: Chinese

Before height: Under 5 feet 2

Shinbone experiment started: *around January 2006.*

Current height growth from shinbone routine: 5 feet 4.5 inch in less than 5 months *(grown more than 2.5 inches)*

Mom's height: 5' 2".

Dad's height: 5'5"

Location: California *(USA)*

Summary: Jeff, on average grew about 0.25 to 0.5 cm every week.

His growth was very rapid and consistent because he goes beyond no man has ever gone before – running and sprinting like a mad man!

What did Jeff do?

In Jeff's own words…

"1. Run at top speed on the concrete street for about 20-30 min. This may be difficult at first because it is hard to keep at top speed for that long period of time.

But it's important that you run at top speed because it will release a huge amount of GH.

If you don't believe me, ask any doctor or look it up".

MONTH ONE:

week one:

I ran three miles a day without stopping in less than 26 minutes.

I was short, slow, and I wasn't the most athletic person in my class.

On top of that, I had really short legs so it was pretty hard for me to run this fast.

. I didn't grow at all so I got angry and tried harder.

week two (aka The Hell):

I ran around four miles a day in around half an hour. The training was really killing me.

My grade dropped from all A's to 4 A's and 2 B's.

I didn't do most of my homework and I didn't really care about school.

All I wanted to do was eat and sleep.

It was like hell to push myself to run every day.

Once I ran so hard, I felt blood come up to my throat. I'm not even joking about this.

I came home and started spitting in the bathroom.

My spit was red and it scared me. But I just kept on going and going.

week three:

Three weeks of torture and still no progress was a big disappointment.

I knew I was doing something wrong and I had better change it fast. I went on the internet, read some books, talked to a few doctors, and basically did a little research.

I found out that the best way to increase your hormone level is to do short and intense exercise rather than long ones.

I also found out that if you don't stretch out the microfractures you made, the bone will get thicker but not longer.

MONTH TWO

week one:

Actually, it was probably the first weeks of month two that I've noticed growth.

It was around the end of the first month and the beginning of the second month when a miracle began happening.

I went to church, prayed God, and changed my routine to fast and intense exercises followed by a method of stretching out microfractures.

I used to tape dumb bells to my leg which was effective but extremely uncomfortable.

I would run for about five to seven minutes at my maximum sprinting pace, rest for about ten to fifteen minutes (I was so tired.

I was going to pass out, seriously) and run for another five minutes.

The speed and intensity of the run is far more important than the amount of time you spend running, as I have learned the hard way.

According to doctors and experts, the intensity of my training had enabled me to produce about 400% more growth hormone than normal jogging would have offered.

I believe the reason most people fail to grow with running is because they don't do it hard enough.

After the run I would go home, drink milk, stretch, sleep with weights taped on my leg, and the combination of 400% GH from exercise, microfractures that're stretched out by weight, deep quality sleep from being exhausted, and the calcium from milk had enabled me to grow one solid cm by the end of the week.

Now that I know how to grow taller, I kept on running each night at a faster and faster pace for a shorter amount of time.

week two:

I will run at super speed for about 30 seconds, walk for a minute or two, and then run again at super speed.

I was surprised that I can keep up with the cars driving on the local street.

Even though I can only keep up with them for about half a minute, it was still a good indication that I was running at a pretty good pace.

I began enjoying this training. I was addicted to the rush of hormone that followed each run.

I grew another .75 cm by the end of the week.

Since I always measure myself at night, I know the height I gained is solid.

week three:

Picked up a pair of ankle weights after visiting a sports store.

MONTH THREE:

week one:

My legs are beginning to hurt.

First the muscles, then the bones. I would often pull a few muscles each night and it really hurts.

My friends are beginning to notice my new height. I lied to them and said that it must've been a late growth spurt because I know they are too dumb to understand what's really happening.

The compliments keep me going. I was more than three inches shorter than my dad and now I am only about an inch or so shorter.

I grew about 1 1/4 inches in these three months and I was on fire.

week two:

Muscle pain got better but the bone pain got worse.

It hurts to walk and I can seriously feel the microfractures in my leg from all that hard-concrete pounding.

I decided to ignore the pain. Big mistake. When I measured this weekend, I shrank a little.

I did a little research and decided that the newly formed bone must be compressing from the running.

I decided to listen to my body and take time to heal the microfractures before continuing the routine.

week three:

Switched from high intensity running to swimming.

Swimming helps me further increase the production of GH while stretching and healing my bones.

MONTH FOUR:

Resting and healing the microfractures has given me close to two permanent inches. I know it's permanent because I always measure at night when I'm the shortest.

MONTH FIVE

I stopped swimming and now I'm back into running, fracturing my bones, and healing my bone. My leg bones are now a lot thicker and longer.

I moved from a size 12 regular pant to a size 14 regular pant and from 8 to 8.5 pair of shoes.

I now stand about the same height as my father, which is pretty incredible because only a few months ago, I was considerably shorter than him.

Well, that's my story. If I keep going at this speed, I should get to 5' 7" by the end of the year, no problem.

The year after that I'll be like 5' 11".

The point is to keep the progress consistent.

One thing I learned is that you should learn to listen to your heart and your body.

If your heart tells you to do whatever it takes to make a truly special girl really happy, then you should listen to it and die for her.

If your body tells you that you should take a few weeks to heal your microfractures, you should do it.

To answer your question, the height seems very proportional so far. But I'll get you some pictures soon and you be the judge.

What did his devices look like?

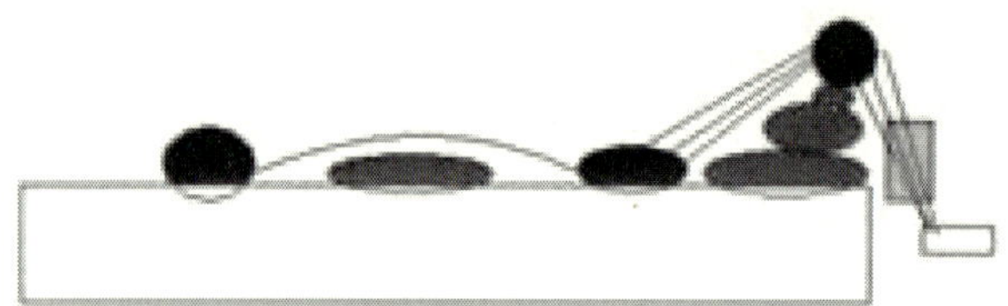

Here's Jeff picture of his sleeping with ankle weight method.

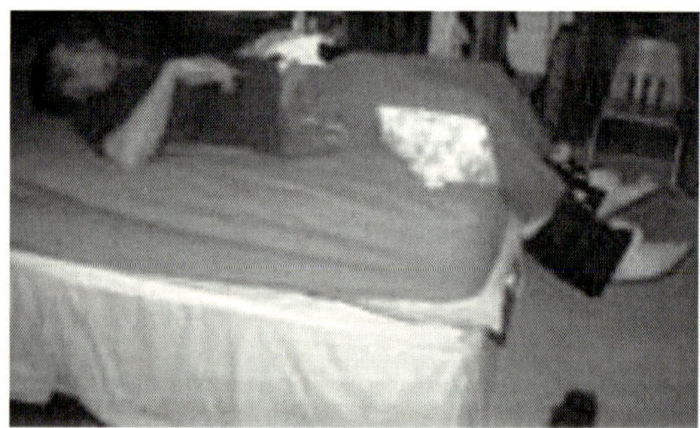

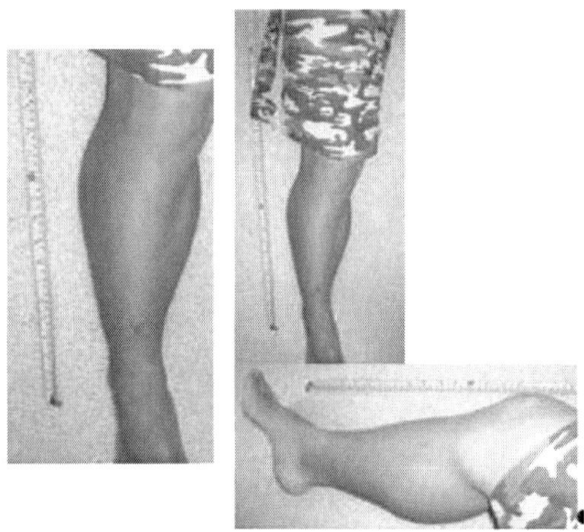

Jeff's after pictures *(2 inches taller than before) ...* there are no before pictures.

"I stopped growing a year or two ago and my recent growth has been very rapid – 0.25 to 0.5 cm every week. I've grown a total of 2.5 inches in the legs within 5 months. Whether it's a growth spurt or not, there is a very REAL connection between my INTENSE routine and recent growth. Read my story very carefully and then draw your conclusion." **– Jeff**

EVAN'S REVISED AND IMPROVED ANKLE WEIGHTS ROUTINE.

"Good day,

Of course, I will not disclose my real name, so let's just believe it is Evan Svensson.

I am male, just turned 23, and have been doing the shinbone routine for approximately three months.

While I saw absolutely no results at first, I realized I was not creating sufficient microfractures.

I was relying on my gym routine to create them and found out that it was not enough.

In fact, cycling and such doesn't create any since there's no impact, despite that it is good exercise for the legs, and could even help them in the effort.

At this time, I started my own separate routine specifically for shin bone growth.

I jog, in place, in my room with 5 kgs of ankle weights for 30-60 minutes, between moderate and fast pace, making sure my feet hit the ground strongly.

Then I immediately sit (lying down, actually) with around 25 pounds strapped to my legs for 1-2 hours, then I go to sleep, without standing until the morning.

I don't sleep with the ankle weights on though, I can't get used to it.

Two weeks ago, I measured (at about 10:30 at night) at 5'10" exactly, then the next week 5'10" and 1/8, then today 5'10" and 1/4.

I even feel a bit taller in relation to everyone else.

What has me baffled is that I am 95% percent certain that I grew 1/4 an inch in the past two weeks, now that I properly modified the routine.

How does that happen with only a quarter inch??? And I think the routine did this because my shins definitely look a little bit longer.

This really gives me hope because if I continue at this rate, I could theoretically gain several inches over the next year or two.

My goal is to gain around 3", but if I could get more than that, I will try hard to do so.

In fact, I think I could start growing at a faster rate if I ramp up the intensity of the jogging.

I actually feel the sensation of my shin bones being "pushed out" or stretched from the inside sometimes, and it feels strange, did Jeff report this?

Well, I have said a lot, and the only reason I am writing to tell you guys all this is because I am convinced the shin bone routine works.

It doesn't mean it is a miracle technique, but again, I am sure of it that it causes growth.

Ouch, was Jeff disappointed? I don't know, I'd be pretty happy with a 2.5" gain, but I'm a lot taller than him.

However, I don't see why most people can't gain something substantial with a combination of leg and spine growth and a lot of work.

But to answer your questions, yes, I jog with 10 pounds on each leg, and sit with 25 pounds on each leg afterward, then I sleep after that without standing, to keep the microfractures from compressing before they have 8 hours or so to heal.

I take multivitamins and drink more milk than most people, but I don't think that alone does anything for height.

I think's it's necessary to keep from being perpetually exhausted.

I don't think you have to compromise your energy to the extreme (as Jeff did) to achieve growth, but time will give me that answer.

But I should probably try adding more weight and sitting with the weights for longer, and jogging for longer as well.

I think longer duration does create more microfractures which is always a good thing in the way of this technique.

But, again, I'll find out with time. I'll contact you if/when I hit the 1/2" mark. Thanks.

Just letting you know, you told me to contact you guys again when I reached the 1/2" mark, and I measured again yesterday to find that is exactly what has taken place.

I'm pretty sure of it because I measured in the evening, and I was on my feet all day.

I think at this point, there's still no telling what is causing this, but I have concluded that I am growing about 1/8 an inch every week.

I've yet to get myself to grow faster, but I am working on that at the moment.

My goal is to reach 6'0" by the fall, but I am hoping I can surpass that, even. If you have any questions, let me know.

I'll give you all the information you need, but to answer question one, I do not have any before pictures, but I'm not sure if it is time to send in after pictures just yet, why don't we wait, once again until about September or October, because I am fairly convinced that I will have achieved substantial growth since then.

If I do decide to submit any pictures, it will be of the legs only, for privacy reasons.

The legs already look significantly longer after just 1/2" so if I manage to pick up 2 or 3 inches in all, the length of the shins as seen in the photos won't lie,

If you study the proportions of people, you'll see that most people's lower legs are not that long, even those above 6'.

Suggesting the shin bone might be the little-known window for height increase.

To answer question 2, my original height is 5'10", I'm Male, around 151lbs, I live in New Haven, Connecticut. I'm 23 years old, and Caucasian (of English descent to be precise).

My current height is 5'10" and a half, in light of my recent routine. My goal is to reach 6'0" by the fall of this year, which I think is doable, but with a combination of leg and spine growth, I'm actually hoping to be around 6'3" within five years, but that is a big undertaking, not so sure that could happen.

In short, I am convinced I am growing around 1/8" every week, since around March 3 or so, when I modified the routine to be more effective. My mother is around 5'3", my father is 6'1".

I must note that I am not entirely sure that my growth plates are closed. Though I have not grown naturally since I was around 20.

I still have the face and body of a teen; I'm actually routinely mistaken for a 16-year-old.

The reason I mention all this, is because it suggests my bones aren't all that mature yet, that probably bears some significance in my case.

But one thing I can say is that I am fairly sure my newfound growth was in the shins, they look decidedly longer, and somehow.

I feel I can run a little bit faster on the treadmill now, you aspiring runners might want to keep that in mind.

After reading Jeff's story through and through, I decided to change the routine to ensure many microfractures are created and that they are stretched out while they are "fresh".

My routine is as follows:

1.) Jog for around 30-60 minutes with 5kgs of ankle weights attached to EACH LEG. Take a 1-2-minute break about once every 10-15 minutes.

It all depends on how athletic you are.

I, being quite active, could handle it, but please, don't hurt yourself, such action is NOT NECESSARY to achieve growth (I'll get to that later).

2.) Take five to ten minutes to make so your night regimen is done.

3.) Strap 25 pounds of ankle weights to EACH LEG, and lie down with the legs extended over the bed front bedpost and stay that way for 1-2 hours.

If it starts to feel a bit intolerable after about 50 minutes, I think it is a sure sign it is working.

But don't allow yourself to suffer extreme pain, sometimes,

I try taking the weights off for ten minutes, then going another hour before sleeping. It pays to have a high bed, by the way, get one if you can.

Mine is almost four feet off the ground.

And it helps, if your legs touch the ground at all, it will hurt your progress because it provides some relief from the weight.

IMPORTANT:

It is imperative that you do not stand once you start the final process, not until the next morning.

I discovered this point from Jeff who stated that once you step on the ground again, the microfractures compress back down, and thus, you're no better off than when you started jogging.

Make sure your remotes are with you so you can turn the TV, DVD, surround sound, etc. off when you are ready to go to sleep.

I'll finally close with this: try not to tell everyone you know about this routine, I've told no one besides you guys. I mean, if EVERYONE is tall, is height so great?

THE IDEAL ANKLE WEIGHTS PROGRAM OR WORK PLAN.

9 pm: *Begin jogging with 5 kg ankle weights for 40 minutes to create microfractures.*

9:40 pm: *Finished jogging. Take a few minutes to rest and immediately get ready to stretch out the microfractures by sitting or lying down with ankle weights.*

9:45 pm: *Begin sitting or lying down with 5kg for 1 hour non-stop.*

10:45 *pm: Finished sitting/ lying with ankle weights? Take an 8-minute break to restore normal blood circulation from the legs to the body.*

Do NOT walk or stand.

10:55 pm: *Resume sitting or lying down with ankle weights for 40 minutes non-stop.*

11:35 pm: *Finished sitting/lying with ankle weights? Go to sleep immediately to allow the stretched microfractures to heal and recover.*

Do NOT stand or walk around because you may compress the shinbone.

After creating so much microfractures by sitting with ankle weights, you may experience some "stretching" sensations in your lower legs

C. LEG LENGTHENING WITH JUMPING SUCCESS STORY

Jieyagsen's Jumping routine.

In his own words...

"Hi guys, today I want to share with you guys about my story for growing taller.

I was so obsessed with growing taller.

*I searched online all over, but all I got were bull sh*t!*

It was just stretching all day long... even though that does make you grow like a cm after all the pain for pulling your legs for a year.

*That won't get me to 6'0 for Sh*t!*

And they even told you something like (your height is pre-determined by your gene from your parent and also exercise won't going to make you taller).

It likes telling you're doomed!! you can't do anything it at all, just embrace it. I mean screwed that man...

So, I was 5'6 when I was 17, From 14 to 17 I only grew 4 cm, which means 1 cm annually.

And I slept very late at night at around 3am. So, I decided to change all of my bad habit, sleep before 11 pm, no masturbating (masturbating will cause your bone to fuse and mature faster).

Also, I started Running and Touching Sky!

I started running for 30 mins, and "Touching Sky" which is jump as high as possible, arm trying to reach something beyond your reach.

(imagine like you are jumping up trying to touch the basketball backboard) jump 100-200 times a day (Jump with full force).

I continued this exercise for entire 2 years every single day it was very rough, my leg and shoulder hurt a lot.

But I grew 7 inches!!!!!!!like you just have to be consistent,

It's not like you will grow 7 inches just overnight, it's the fact that you have to keep doing every day!!

I'm currently 19 standing at 6'1, I'll push to 6'2.

How does this work? So Running is most basic and effective exercise.

Plus, it is a full body workout and it releases human growth hormone to boost your height, it just makes your body fit overall.

But the most important exercise is Jumping.

Ever wonder why people who play basketball are usually taller?

Because when you are jumping, the gravity is pulling your entire body down, so it is a natural stretch.

Touching Sky" is even more effective and better than playing basketball, because even when you play basketball you won't jump as much as just pure full burst jumping.

Think of it as concentrated exercise that you jumped more, and much higher, so the result is also concentrated in one spot!

Also, you can run and jump anywhere, anytime, no money to be spent.

Be sure to sleep before 11 pm though, because it was important, if not all your exercise will be done in vain.

I was just inspired by one of my 21-year-old friend who also grew taller by 6 inches.

Just be consistent and exercise every day., You will grow taller in no time. PEACE OUT!

CHAPTER 6

COMMON MISTAKES TO AVOID

(Steps to take to grow taller after puberty)

1. Not stretching on a Daily Basis.

When you add a couple of inches to your torso, you may think it's time to rest with your inches in your pocket. Poof! All Your gains will disappear in thin air.

You will start feeling shorter than normal as time passes by. I've mentioned it a couple of times, that height gained in torso isn't permanent but stabilizing it is very simple.

Just watch your posture, perform the stretches in the advanced stage routine every day before stepping out, and do the sit ups.

All this may be done within 5 minutes or less every morning before stepping out yet it will make you feel better.

If you're in a rush, then just hang for 30 seconds and do 5 to 10 sit ups. Your torso height will be stable all day.

2. Inconsistency

This is one of the biggest yet most common challenges that will hinder your progress.

In most cases, inconsistency may not be an option but since these exercises are time consuming, you may have other priorities that may derail you during the course of the routine.

If you are following the routine one week then off for a week or two, don't expect results.

That's why I suggested, you clear time say a month or two to fully focus on the routine or make height increase a priority in your life.

This will allow you to notice any slight mistake that may be hindering your progress. The mistakes are many, yet any one or two of them are enough to affect the results.

3. Not keeping your mouth shut

Don't go telling every Tom, Dick and Harry about your goal of increasing height especially if you're past puberty.

Not only will you be scoffed at ninety percent of the time, a study conducted at New York University found that blabbing about your goals can give you a false sense of accomplishment, making you less likely to actually go after achieving them.

But at least tell your girlfriend, right? Nope.

"By not telling anyone, you're making sure that your goal is something you're really doing for yourself," says K.C. McCulloch, PhD, an assistant professor at Idaho State University who worked on the study.

You won't run the risk of letting anyone else's opinions get in your way if you keep your mouth shut.

"What stops a lot of people from doing the things they dream of is other people," says Susan B. Wilson, a life coach in Michigan and founder of Get Over It, Move On!

"If you tell someone you want to apply to a graduate program, they may go on about how terrible the campus is... and you may start to believe them when you really should be trusting your own gut."

Beyond that, loved ones may have ulterior motives for being naysayers.

If you announce that you're going to be devoting tons of time to a big goal, a good friend or your significant other may worry that he or she will see less of you and subconsciously distract you from the finish line.

Doing something just for you feels selfish in a really good way. "Women tend to overextend themselves for loved ones," says psychologist *Lucy Jo Palladino, PhD, author of Find Your Focus Zone. "So, if you can have something that is yours, it can feel really special."*

4. Not having enough G.H released by the body.

Some folks try the cycling method, ankle Weights or the stretches independently hoping to get results.

Without G.H, you may luckily grow slightly but you will miss out on the intrinsic value of G.H.

It is simply the fountain of growth.

I already mentioned how chaos training was the turning point of my grow taller campaign.

so, the role of G.H can't be emphasized more.

Research though shows that most G.H is released after Weight lifting, H.I. I. E and during sleep. You may fast as well but not every day and I personally never relied on fasting for long so, I don't have much experience with it.

For most females though, fasting may be an option if you are avoiding weights or for some reason can't sprint.

5.Not including abdominal work -outs in your Routine

Again, stretching alone without abdominal work-outs is a waste of energy.

At one point, I decided to throw abdominal exercises out of my grow taller exercise routine thinking they were wasting my time.

I lost almost all the height I had gained in the torso in a very short time.

I regained my height in torso just after a week of

reincorporating the sit-ups on a daily basis.

You may go a day or two without these workouts but please don't abandon them for good.

6. Not having enough Quality sleep on a regular basis.

According to scientists from the *University of Wisconsin*, at least 90% of bone growth occurs at night.

Sleep is vital for healing, repair and recovery.

Your muscles will become rigid and you will end up losing a couple of inches if you're always fatigued.

Ignore your sleeping posture and focus on the quality of sleep with whatever posture.

If you have a problem attaining slow wave sleep,

then ensure you go to bed by latest mid night.

Initially, it may be challenging to adjust but, in a few days, your circadian rhythm or internal clock will be adjusted and you will be able to adjust.

If getting sleep is a problem, then try taking a cup of warm milk before going to bed and you will sleep like a baby.

Your body requires a fatigue and stress-free environment to continuously grow after puberty.

Pro tip:

If you fail to catch sleep during the middle of the night, (at least for some reason this happens to all of us once in a while).

Don't rush to return to or force sleep. Stay awake for at least 30 minutes unless you feel very sleepy.

You will experience another spike in G.H released and you won't feel as lethargic as you would if you returned to sleep before the 25 – 30-minutes mark. G.H released during sleep helps to recuperate the body.

7. Doing chaos exercises more than twice a week.

When you're just beginning, desperation kicks in and you want fast results.

You may think that by spiriting or doing chaos training more often, more G.H will be released and you will get quick results. But this is counterproductive. There's nothing you will do to force your body to grow faster. Growth is a process.

So, doing chaos training exercises very often will instead stunt your body and you will end up not getting results.

I don't advise you to fast very often as well.

Less is more when it comes to this.

Unfortunately, I learnt this the hard way after wasting a lot of time.

The law of diminishing returns applies here.

Every first time in the week you do chaos training,

more growth hormones will be released and the amount released reduces as you continue doing chaos exercises.

Most G.H is released when Chaos training is done spontaneously shocking thc body to rclease lactic acid for muscle recovery. Lactic acid then triggers G.H release. Do chaos training more frequently, then the body becomes accustomed and less lactic acid will be released.

In fact, your body also needs ample time to recover from these chaos exercises.

8. being pessimistic

This is another major challenge. In fact, if you have doubts that you will make it, I advise you to work on your mindset otherwise this will not work for you.

Everything begins with your brain. The moment you begin doubting what you are doing, not only will you lack the zeal to follow the routine, you may even doubt any gains you may achieve.

Staying positive is extremely critical here. If you're below average height, staying positive may not be a problem since you may be facing a number of challenges with your stature and the only option is to keep trying until you make it.

Even minor gains will excite you and you'll be optimistic and positive which is a recipe for success in any field.

Those who are above average don't know what it means to be too short so, there's plenty of room for pessimism.

9. Ignoring the Role of hydration.

I already discussed how staying dehydrated for long may shrink the discs in the back bone.

In fact, every time your body is dehydrated, you feel shorter than normal.

Keeping your body hydrated will have the opposite impact on the discs which will make you slightly taller.

In addition; According to sports nutrition expert Dr. John Berardi, your muscles won't grow to their maximum potential if you don't drink enough water.

10. Measuring your height very often to check your progress.

Every time you measure your height and you find yourself at the same height or even shorter, it elicits negative emotions.

You will be pessimistic and feel like you're wasting your time which will dampen your spirits.

You will stand against your Wall mounted height

rod every morning and evening hours to check if

you are progressing, sometimes finding yourself shorter which will be depressing.

This will psychologically impact the way you work-out.

Measure your height only once or twice a week and the little progress you will have made will be enough to motivate you.

11. Abandoning your posture

This is one of the biggest mistakes especially when it comes to sitting posture.

Problem is, we spend plenty of time seated. Be it working, watching a movie or T.V or even reading.

Just imagine how much height you lose in the torso if you spend hours compressing the spinal discs.

Most spinal disc compression occurs with upright sitting and sitting in a slouched position.

Pro tip:

The harder the surface you sit on, the easier it will be to compress the spine and lose torso height.

So, use chairs or seats with zig zag springs so you stop worrying about your sitting posture.

The springs in the chair act as shock absorbers taking almost all your weight off your spine. Your torso height will be more stable when you utilize such chairs or seats.

Supplementary Mistakes

1. Not including milk and amino Acid rich proteins regularly not necessarily every day. Amino acid supplements may also do the job.

2. Jumping rope, and kicking out are easy and cheap but not very efficient and not chaotic exercises, so they just eat into your time.

3. Not including long walks two to three times a week especially if you want to lengthen legs.

4. Sprinting on treadmills isn't as effective as running on a hard surface. So, avoid sprinting on treadmills at all costs just because you may miss out on bone thickening, and microfractures which are created by the stamping impact of sprinting on a hard surface.

If you must use a treadmill because of weather, then just set the incline to at least level 1.

5. Avoid carrying heavy loads on your back. Especially backpacks.

6. If you are a Weight lifter, utilize the days of chaos training otherwise you may first prioritize height increase before muscle building.

Summary of Steps to Take to Grow Taller After Puberty

1. Stretch Regularly.

2. Ensure you increase your body's ability to release growth hormones naturally.

3. Include a few abdominal workouts in your routine but regularly.

4. Ensure you have a good comfortable 8 hours of sleep.

5. Keep your mouth shut

6. Watch your posture

7. Don't do chaos training more than twice a week.

8. If you're pessimistic, this isn't for you.

9. Ensure you hydrate very often

CHAPTER 7

DAILY MEAL PLAN

You will need a simple to follow yet efficient regular meal plan that will include all the essential nutrients for growth at every meal and snack.

This will ensure that you'll naturally have less room for nutrient-poor choices *(in soft drinks, chips, candy, desserts and alike.)* that don't contribute anything to body growth.

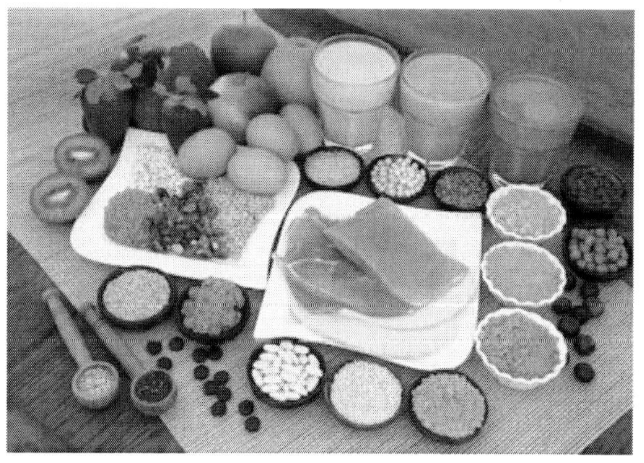

The most essential foods and nutrients to be included in your meals include;

Milk – For growth factor 1, calcium, and proteins

Animal meats – Meat and pork for zinc, poultry for high quality proteins rich in amino acids.

Eggs – For high quality proteins, minerals and up to 13 different vitamins especially vitamin A and D.

Tinned fish – For Vitamin A, B1, B2, B3, B5, B6, B12, D and E not to forget calcium if fish has bones.

Potatoes – For vitamin C, potassium, magnesium, iron, copper and manganese and most B vitamins.

Broccoli – Source of Vitamins A, B9, C, and K.

Oats – For protein, fiber and lots of minerals necessary for bone development like manganese, magnesium, zinc, folate and iron.

Soy beans – For quality proteins with plenty of amino acids, zinc, vitamin C, calcium, manganese, potassium, and several B vitamins.

Whole wheat bread- For fiber and proteins.

Nuts and Seeds – For vitamins, proteins, healthy fats, fiber, minerals such as magnesium, potassium, calcium, plant iron and zinc.

Plenty of fruits and **water.**

* Begin your day with a fruit say an apple, a banana or any of other nutritious fruit.

*Then when it comes to the main breakfast, you may choose to have cereal(oats), Greek yoghurt, eggs, seeds and nuts, or whole wheat bread.

If you decide cereal, organic whole grain oatmeal will be a good option. whole grain Oats and bread contain plenty of soluble fiber.

This type of fiber dissolves in water and tends to slow the movement of food through the digestive system.

*If you chose whole grain cereal, it may be an opportunity for you to add low-fat milk.

Anywhere between 250ml - 500ml will do.

*If you choose bread, you may have it with a couple of hard-boiled eggs, nuts or even seeds.

Egg whites contain amino-acid rich proteins while the yolks contain Vitamin A, D as well as other minerals like calcium, magnesium, potassium, iron, and zinc.

*Otherwise, you may throw anything into the mix for breakfast.

*Take half a liter *(500mls)* of water first thing in morning. I know it sounds ridiculous to some of you but once you get used, you will like it.

Take another half a liter at once 15 – 30 minutes after your main breakfast and half a liter after lunch and supper.

That's 2 liters of water a day.

You've just met at least 80% of your daily requirement of 2.5 – 3 liters a day.

You can rehydrate every time you take a leak to hit the target of 2.5 liters.

Your body and brain will get on the knees and thank you so much.

*The time when you have your meals may not count much since that may depend on circumstances.

*If you wish to have snacks, between main meals, snacking on soy or seeds like pumpkin seeds and other nuts like peanuts will be a good idea.

You may even slot in other fruits like avocadoes which are rich in zinc and healthy fats.

*When it comes to lunch and Dinner, you may throw anything into the mix as long as it facilitates body growth.

Lean Meat, Poultry, Fish, Beans, vegetables, potatoes, whole grain rice, whole grain pasta, fruit juices and alike.

*If you have a special weekend diet, the paleo diet will be the best option.

Use the nutrition chapter as a guide when deciding what to eat and when. At the end of the day, you may require no supplements.

The main pointers here are;

- Take at least 2-3 liters of water every day.

- Two glasses (500mls) of low-fat milk every day.

- Stock up on pumpkin seeds or other zinc-rich fruits, seeds and nuts.

- You may snack on them anytime during the day.

- Broccoli, and other cruciferous vegetables should feature very often on your menu.

- Consume animal meats particularly poultry and fish at least three times during the week, as well as eggs.

- If you're vegetarian, Quinoa and soy will be good options.

CHAPTER 8

FINDOUT WHICH SECTION OF YOUR BODY IS GROWING

As discussed earlier, your body has the potential to grow in the neck, thoracic, abdominal, and lumbar areas.

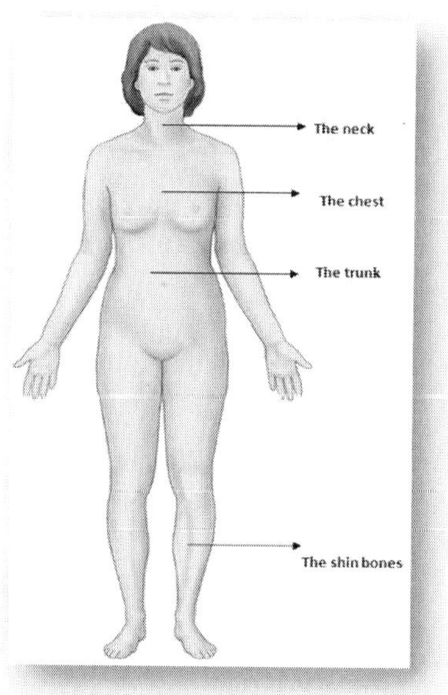

If you intend to increase height in both legs and torso, it's imperative to take measurements for each section to know where you are progressing or falling short.

This is very important because your daily workout routine involves all these areas so, you may for instance gain an aggregate height of 2 inches without knowing where exactly the growth is coming from.

This may be your target, but then your body may look out of proportion.

Hence, note somewhere if necessary, your before height.

I used to do so in the beginning.

The neck and chest.

Place The metal tip at the end of your tape measure on the top of your head and run out the tape to the point where the chest ends which is just below your chest.

You may combine the chest and neck because the aggregate increase in height in these areas isn't likely to be more than an inch.

The abdominal area (trunk)

Measure from just below the chest to just above your groin. Growth in this section is likely to contribute a significant if not the most height of up to 1 to 3 inches with the aid of the stretches, inflatable cushion and abdominal workouts.

The shin bones.

Growth in shin bones may contribute 1 – 3 inches depending on time invested.

Simply take measurements from the middle of your knee joint to the bottom of tour foot.

If your knees are fleshy, finding a spot to mark may be a challenge otherwise there's a slight dip between the knee joint area when you look at the inside of your leg.

Take measurements from that line to the bottom of your foot.

Ways to Measure your Height

There are different ways you can measure your height.

You can use a tape measure, divide the body into three parts as illustrated above then you add up the measurements to get your aggregate height.

Alternatively, you can stand against a wall probably one of your bedroom walls and mark your before height then check again after a week or two and see the difference between before and after to know your progress.

I grew with a bit of consistency so, every four months I expected some progress. You may also experience the same.

Hence, checking on a weekly basis shouldn't only be for progress, but also to find if you are losing some height and if that's the case, then based on the checklist discussed below, you may need to do something about it.

Finally, a digital stadiometer may accurately do the job.

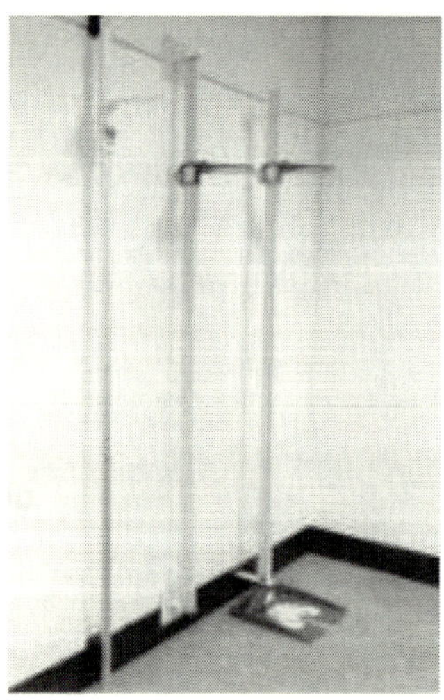

WHY YOUR HEIGHT MAY FLUCTUATE THROUGHOUT THE DAY BY UP TO AN INCH.

First of all, as mentioned earlier, DO NOT check your progress very often.

Secondly, your height will never be stable while performing stretching exercises due to the following circumstances;

a) Very early in the morning hours before breakfast, you will be taller than normal.

b) Moments after eating, your height reduces slightly in most cases.

c) After long walks, exercising or when the entire body is exhausted, you will be slightly shorter.

Some report losing up to 1- 2 inches.

d) When you are dehydrated, your muscles will shrink making you a little shorter.

e) When you don't have enough sleep, you may be shorter the day after especially when fatigued.

f) When you go a couple of days without doing sit ups or the stretches, you may lose some height.

g) After spending too much time seated especially on a hard surface, you will be shorter.

h) Last but not least, according to Elizabeth Lombardo Ph.D., a psychologist and physical therapist at Wexford Pennsylvania, Stress affects our musculoskeletal system, resulting in tight, contracting muscles and spasms which makes you lose an inch or two. Thus, when you're stressed, you may be shorter than normal.

A number of variables will affect your height throughout the day hence when you find yourself shorter than expected, don't panic or be distressed. Stay calm and try to find the possible culprit.

This happened to me several times during the course of the routine and I know how distressing and demoralizing it can be to find yourself an inch or two shorter.

What I noticed is; the best time to measure your height is late in evening long after lunch but before dinner.

CHAPTER 10

HEALTH CONDITIONS THAT AFFECT BODY GROWTH

As mentioned earlier, body growth and development is influenced by both natural and environmental factors.

Ill health contributes to the natural factors.

Health conditions that may affect body growth include but are not limited to;

1. Arthritis

when children develop joint inflammation, growth of the nearby bones is often affected.

If it occurs before age 3, the affected limb may be longer than expected, but if it occurs after age 9,

the growth plates may close earlier than expected, leading to reduced leg length.

2. Anemia

The blood is made up of red blood cells, white blood cells, platelets, and plasma.

The predominant cells in the blood are the red blood cells whose primary function is to supply oxygen and nutrients to the body's cells and to remove waste products.

The red blood cells can transport oxygen because they contain hemoglobin, a complex protein that contains iron.

Anemia results when the number of red blood cells is reduced below normal, or if there is a decrease in the amount of the body's hemoglobin.

The most common cause of anemia in children and adolescents is iron deficiency.

Iron is essential for all tissues in a young child's developing body.

Adolescent girls may be at risk due to their irregular eating habits (caused by concerns about body image) compounded by normal menstrual blood loss.

3. Growth Hormone abnormalities

Children with reduced growth hormone have a much-reduced growth spurt around the time of puberty, leading to short stature.

Conversely, if excessive growth hormone is present before growth plates close, "giantism" a dramatic increase in height — may follow.

4. Hypogonadism

This condition is marked by a reduction in sex hormones, including testosterone and estrogen. Affected persons may have little or no growth spurt at the time puberty is expected.

5. IMAGe syndrome

This is characterized by the association of Intrauterine *(inside uterus)* growth retardation, metaphyseal, hip abnormalities, short limbs as well as Genital anomalies.

A gene mutation thought to be linked to large stature has been pinpointed as the culprit of IMAGe syndrome.

Children with IMAGe syndrome have stunted growth before birth hence they end up with a smaller-than-normal body and organs.

Complications from the disease can be life-threatening.

6. Hypothyroidism

A condition where your thyroid gland does not make enough thyroid hormone.

A reduction in the normal amount of thyroid hormone during childhood typically leads to short stature among other problems such as; poor school performance, fatigue, constipation and cold intolerance7. Osteoporosis

A reduction in the normal amount of thyroid hormone during childhood typically leads to short stature among other problems such as poor school performance, fatigue, constipation and cold intolerance.

7. Osteoporosis

A condition that causes bones to weaken and become so brittle or fragile to the point that fractures can so easily occur.

People tend to lose height as they age mainly due to osteoporosis and reduced water content in the disks *(so that the distance between each vertebra is reduced).*

On average, women lose about 2 inches over their lifetime, while men lose about 1 inch.

8. Diabetes

A group of metabolic disorders in which there's a high blood sugar level over a prolonged period.

Symptoms of high blood sugar include frequent urination, increased thirst, and increased hunger.

If left untreated, diabetes can cause many complications.

Diabetes that starts during childhood (typically type 1) used to be a common cause of short stature in children, but early recognition and treatment has reduced this effect on height.

9. Cystic fibrosis

A genetic disorder that mainly affects the internal organs like; the lungs, pancreas, intestines, kidneys, and liver.

Long-term issues include difficulty breathing and coughing up mucus.

Poor linear growth and inadequate weight gain are very common problems among children suffering from cystic fibrosis.

The most important factors involved in growth failure are malnutrition, chronic inflammation, lung disease, and corticosteroid treatment.

10. Kidney failure

Researchers have found that many factors cause growth failure in children with chronic kidney disease.

In addition to removing wastes and extra fluid from the blood, the kidneys perform important functions for a child's growth.

Damaged kidneys can slow a child's growth by;

a) Causing mineral and bone disorder, which occurs when vitamin D is not turned into calcitriol, which starves the bones of calcium.

b) Phosphorus levels rise in the blood and draw calcium out of the bones and into the blood, causing the bones to weaken thereby creating an imbalance of sodium, potassium, and acid-base levels in the blood, also called acidosis.

When blood is not balanced, the body slows growth to focus energy on restoring the balance.

TREATMENTS THAT MAY AFFECT BODY GROWTH.

Asthma inhalers

Research, conducted by the federal university of Rio Grande in Brazil and university of Montreal in Canada, showed that children who used steroids for asthma had slower growth rates compared to those not using the medications.

The report goes on to suggest that children treated daily with inhaled corticosteroids may grow approximately half a centimeter less during the first year of treatment."

Glucocorticoids

Medicines that reduce inflammation and used to treat a number of illnesses in children like allergies and asthma.

Such medicines include; cortisone, hydrocortisone and beclomethasone among others.

A high-dose of such drugs affects bone formation which leads to growth failure in children.

ADHD medication

Attention-deficit hyperactivity disorder (ADHD) is a mental disorder characterized by problems paying attention, excessive activity, or difficulty controlling behavior which is not appropriate for a person's age.

According to a recent study published in the Medical Journal of Australia today, adolescent boys with attention deficit hyperactivity disorder are more likely to be shorter than their same-age peers.

According to the study, prolonged treatment with stimulant medication for more than three years was associated with a slower rate of physical development during puberty yet the symptoms never reduced.

Short term treatment is therefore recommended since the benefits outweigh the risks.

CHAPTER 10

THE POWER OF YOUR MIND

"There are no limitations to the mind except those we acknowledge and Whatever the mind of man can conceive and believe, it can achieve" - ***Napoleon Hill***

Your mind will play a central role when it comes to achieving your objective of height increase.

First of all, you must believe that you will make it. Believing alone will not make you grow tall but it will help you have a positive mind set.

One mistake many make that forces them to give up on their objective of height increase is talking

about it openly.

This has already been discussed further under mistakes to avoid.

Secondly try as much as possible to use imagination. Trust me, it works, though indirectly.

I remember vividly imagining how I would look like with longer legs moments before going to sleep for a couple of days.

Then I started dreaming about it. I experienced one or two dreams in which I was standing taller with longer legs and reflecting on those dreams every morning just kept me all excited and positive.

I started believing that it would happen and finally it did. The other technique I used was to talk to myself aloud while thumping my chest *that "I have to grow taller; I command you my subconscious to tell me how."*

I did so every time I felt low or distressed because of my height and weeks later, I was able to conjure a workout routine that enabled me to achieve my objective.

One thing I've come to learn is that your mind is very powerful and its always ready to hand you solutions to dominating challenges, as long as you're ready to take action.

In most cases, you won't even be aware why you are doing whatever you are doing simply because your subconscious mind is in control.

That's why I insist that being positive is a must.

Your mind won't act if you have doubts or if you are pessimistic. It needs a strong stimulus for it to act in a particular direction.

Auto suggestion, law of attraction, imagination, and faith. All of them work but the moment you have the slightest bit of doubt that you can make it, you will be doomed.

Some say that just by talking to themselves they're able to become taller.

But I don't think self-suggestion automatically makes you taller, rather it prompts your mind to give you the appropriate steps you should take to achieve your goal in form of hunches.

I will leave you with Angel's story picked from one of the forums. I hope it helps...

Re: *My story of growing tall*

« Reply #10 on: November 09, 2011, 11:50:18 PM »Publish

"Hey lovely people,

I grew around 5 to 6 inches tall in 3 months, all thanks to the lovely Universe who responded so quickly to my desire.

I am getting quite some PMs asking me how I did it. So, I thought I will share it in a post here as it will be helpful to anyone who needs it, and anyone can access this even when I am not

online and hence not able to respond to PMs immediately.

I am copy pasting my story, which I just shared with one of our members in a PM.

Before telling you what and how I manifested my desire,

I'll share a small incident with you. It makes me smile every time I think of it.

A couple of days back, my boyfriend's mother came home.

After talking casually for a while, she suddenly exclaimed 'Hey you look really tall. Is it because of your dress?' I said 'No I have grown tall really'.

She kinda made fun of me and said 'Oh ya, right! How can you grow at this age (I am 21 years old)?' I just smiled and said 'It's possible'.

The reason I am telling you this is, most people have preconceived notions about everything,

EVERYTHING! Can you believe that?? They tend to believe that there is a limitation in everything which includes our physical growth.

They also believe that physical growth, especially height, is by large beyond our control. When living in the midst of such people, we also tend to absorb those beliefs subconsciously.

Has this happened to you? It definitely happened to me. So once upon a time, I truly believed that after puberty, girls' growth becomes slow.

And guess what, I actually stopped growing pretty much after puberty! I was 5' 2" and the tallest in class when I was 11 years old (that's when I attained puberty) and by 18 years I was just 5' 3"!!

I hadn't grown more than an inch in 7 years because I believed that was not possible.

Then I learnt about LOA (Law of Attraction) a couple of years ago and started manifesting many things.

Only a few months back, I decided to increase my height with this knowledge. Here is what I did:

I got clear with how tall I wanted to grow. I wanted to be 5' 9". I decided NEVER to think that I am short. If someone commented that I am short I would just ignore it.

I decided not to 'try' to grow tall because then I would just keep attracting 'trying'! So, I started acting 'as if' I am tall. I would just close my eyes and feel nice, proud and confident because of my new height I was about to get into.

I am not very good at visualization so I instead focused on 'feeling' taller rather than 'imagining' myself taller.

Then I did some stretching exercises (which was a part of my dance warm-up sessions anyways) just to convince my mind that I am taking rational steps.

I didn't spend much time exercising though.

That's it.

After a while I totally forgot about growing tall. I got busy with other work and stuff.

Suddenly, people started telling me that I look taller.

So, I checked my height and I was 5'8"!! Just one inch lesser than what I wanted. But now I feel this height is good. 5'9" could have looked a little manly for me. That's my story. Feel free to ask me anything more!"

All the best

Lots of love

Angel

I am living the life of my dreams...NOW

Conclusion

It's quite evident that increasing height after puberty is possible, but many aren't successful because it takes a lot of dedication, patience, self-motivation, initiative, as well as focus to be successful.

This is the reason why desperation plays a significant role. Many are concerned about growth plate's closure, but researchers on this topic concede that the exact mechanism behind epiphyseal fusion is still not completely understood.

Thus, growth plate's closure alone doesn't always mean the end of bone growth.

Bones are always bristling with life and can remodel and grow after puberty which is why cosmetic leg lengthening surgery to individuals who are way past puberty is a success irrespective of growth plate's closure.

DO NOT haste anything hoping for quick results.

Just let everything workout naturally, and the body will play its role of catch up growth.

But most importantly, you may need to clear some time to have your brain and efforts entirely focused on increasing height.

During my first leave of two months, I grew more rapidly than I did during work.

The ball is in your court.

Wish you all the best. Cheers! ◡̈

Made in United States
North Haven, CT
21 March 2025